DELAVIER'S ANATOMY FOR
BIGGER, STRONGER ARMS

FRÉDÉRIC DELAVIER • MICHAEL GUNDILL

DELAVIER'S ANATOMY FOR
BIGGER, STRONGER ARMS

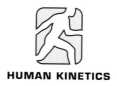

HUMAN KINETICS

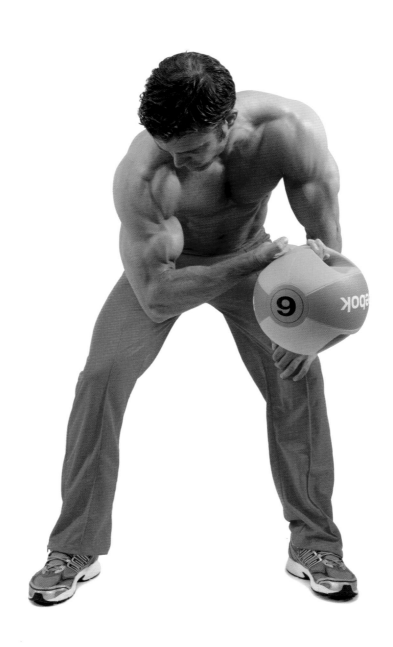

Contents

PART 1
What You Need to Know
Before You Begin 11

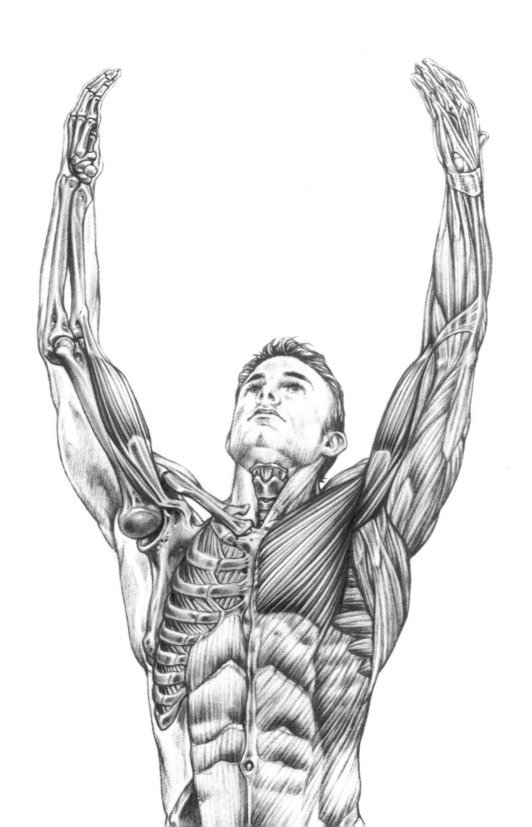

Introduction

When Someone With Huge Arms Talks, Others Listen!

Huge arms evoke power. But in addition to looking good, strong arms give you an unquestionable advantage in many athletic endeavors, such as combat sports, throwing sports, climbing, racket sports, basketball, volleyball, and rowing.

Delavier's Anatomy for Bigger, Stronger Arms relies on this twofold benefit to explain how to develop your arms quickly so they will be
- attractive and impressive as well as
- functional in order to improve your athletic performance.

The programs in this book were developed as a function of
- your goals,
- your schedule,
- your workout equipment, and
- the sport in which you want to improve your performance.

This book is for two groups of people:

1 People who want to create the most effective workout program possible without having to read general strength training manuals that cover every muscle in one book. This book drills down to the essentials by focusing 100 percent on your arms.

2 Athletes who want to enhance their knowledge of the arm muscles in conjunction with using the leading strength training books *The Strength Training Anatomy Workout,* volumes I and II.

What You Need to Know Before You Begin

1 Develop Your Program

20 STEPS TO DEVELOPING YOUR ARM WORKOUT PROGRAM

Developing your workout program relies on fundamental theories that you need to know. Proceeding methodically, we describe the 20 steps that are key to an effective and personalized program.

When you have completed these 20 steps, you will have addressed all possible questions about developing your training program.

1 How should you define your goals?

The very first step in developing an arm workout program is to define your goals well. Are you working out so that you can have arms that are more impressive looking? Or do you want them to be more powerful? Or do you want to improve your athletic performance?

You most likely have several goals. However, if you do not define your goals well, then you will find it difficult to set up an optimal program. Write down your goals on paper so that you can read them before every workout. This will help motivate you.

Next, you need to quantify your goals. For example, you want to

- gain half an inch on your arms in 2 months,
- get stronger so you can lift 10 pounds (5 kg) more during curls after 1 month, and

- double the number of sets you can do in 10 minutes so you can increase your endurance in 15 days.

The time frame and how much you hope to achieve should be reasonable and realistic. Keep in mind that no one ever goes as fast as they would like! Quite often, people feel as if they are stalled. However, with a good program, reaching a true plateau is rare. By quantifying your goals and establishing regular and precise steps for achieving those goals, you can more easily measure your progress. Every time you reach a goal, it will motivate you to keep working out.

Standard programs are provided in part 4 of this book. These are only basic plans, and you must personalize them depending on various parameters, which we detail in the following sections.

2 How many arm workouts should you do each week?

Two workouts per week provide an excellent base for your workout program. However, we recommend that beginners do no more than three arm workouts each week. Keep in mind that overtraining is more damaging to your progress than undertraining.

⚠ When you start strength training, you are generally full of enthusiasm and energy. You feel like working out every day so you can make a lot of progress. This much enthusiasm at the beginning could result in decreased strength instead of increased strength (a sure sign of overtraining)! Then you could lose motivation. Results will not happen instantly, so you must learn to be patient.

3 Which days should you work out?

Ideally, you should be able to alternate one day of training with at least one day of rest. Here again, this might not work well with your schedule. In that case, you have to find a balance between the ideal and the feasible:

- **With a program that includes one arm workout per week,** you can choose any day you like.
- **With a program that includes two arm workouts per week,** ideally, those workouts should be spaced out as much as possible, such as Monday and Thursday or Tuesday and Friday. The exception is if you are able to work out only on the weekends. Working the arms two days in a row is not ideal, but you will have the rest of the week to recover.

> ⚠ **Knowing how many times a week to work your arms includes deciding how many rest days to allow between workouts. Muscle grows only during the rest period between workouts and not during the workout itself. It is just as important to rest as it is to work out.**
>
> **If you are not getting stronger from one workout to the next, then it is smart to give your arms more recovery time.**

4 Should you work the biceps and triceps separately?

Normally, you can work the biceps, triceps, and forearms in a single workout. So we recommend working all the muscles of the arm in one workout. Nevertheless, you could always do the biceps and forearms in one workout and do the triceps another day. This is called an advanced split, and we do not recommend it, at least at first.

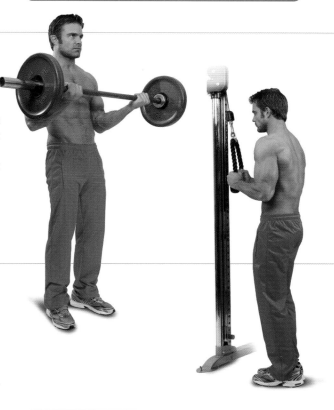

5 What time of day should you work out?

Some people prefer to train in the morning and others in the afternoon or evening. In fact, strength varies depending on the time of day. Some people are stronger in the mornings and weaker in the afternoons. For others, the opposite is true. These fluctuations, due to the central nervous system, are completely normal. It is rare to find people who have consistent strength throughout the day.

Ideally, you should train when your arms are the strongest. The majority of athletes are strongest around 6 to 7 p.m. This works out well since many people are free to exercise at that time.

> ⚠ **Your workout time may be determined by your daily schedule and not by your body. In this case, even if you are not training at the best time for your body, a simple rule is that you should always exercise at the same time each day. Your arms will get used to it and will perform their best at that time.**

6 How many sets of arm exercises should you do for each muscle?

DEFINITION: A set is the total number of repetitions of the same movement done until you reach fatigue.

The volume of work for the arms is determined by two criteria:

1. The number of sets of each exercise
2. The number of exercises per workout

The number of sets is an important factor for muscle growth:

- If you do too few sets, then the muscles will not be stimulated optimally in order to grow rapidly.
- If you do too many sets, then overtraining will prevent the arm muscles from growing.

Your fitness level dictates the number of sets you should do. At first, do no more than 4 sets per muscle.

After 1 month of training, do 5 or 6 sets.
After 2 months of training, do 7 or 8 sets.
After 3 months of training, do 9 or 10 sets.

After 3 months, you will be comfortable choosing your own number of sets based on your arms' needs as well as their capacity for recovery. Still, you should never do more than 30 sets in each arm workout.

 The goal is not to do a bunch of easy sets to reach your target number. It is better to work harder in each set and do fewer total sets than to do the opposite. If you do not have trouble going beyond these maximum limits, it means that your contraction intensity is not high enough. This intensity comes with time and training. Your arms are not able to surpass their limits on a set from one day to the next.

DO NOT FORGET TO WARM UP

The human body is like a car. If you accelerate quickly while the engine is still cold, you will not greatly increase your speed, and you will damage the engine. However, once the engine is warm, a small acceleration will rapidly increase your speed. Like a car, the body's muscles, tendons, and joints work at their optimal level only when they have reached a certain temperature. This is why you must warm up before doing any kind of exercise.

Warming up helps you in three ways:

1. It protects you from injuries.
2. It improves your performance.
3. It helps you mentally prepare for the work you are about to do.

You should always do 1 or 2 light sets as a warm-up before you attempt an exercise with heavy weights. Because these warm-up sets are not very intense, they are not counted as part of the total number of sets discussed previously. **Warning!** The time you spend warming up will vary depending on the seasons and the time of day. For example, in the winter or early morning, your body is colder than in the summer or afternoon, so you need to lengthen your warm-up by 1 or 2 sets. Since you should not shorten the rest of your workout, this means your total workout time will automatically increase.

7 How should you adjust the volume of work?

The number of sets is the first variable to adjust in the volume of work. You should first make changes to this variable, which is a more refined adjustment than just adding exercises. As you become stronger, and when you feel ready, you can add a set here and there.

The best thing is to let your arms tell you how many sets they want to do. The most obvious indicator is when you start to lose strength abnormally from one set to the next. An abrupt loss of strength means that you have perhaps done one set too many. You will know this when you do your next workout.

Obviously, the number of sets that you are able to do can fluctuate from one session to the next. On days when you are feeling great, you might be tempted to add sets. But on days when you are feeling tired, you can reduce the number of sets so that you do not wear yourself out.

You must also keep in mind what you did in the previous workout. If you increased the intensity, the weight, or the number of sets, you must also expect that your recovery time will be longer. This is why a really good workout is often followed by a poor workout. Because you asked more of your arms, their recovery will be more difficult. So that your following workouts do not suffer, it is important to take one day of rest between two workouts.

There is great controversy concerning the number of sets you should do for a muscle. Some say that one very intense set per exercise should suffice. This is true for certain athletes whose central nervous system has the capacity to give its maximum effort for one intense set. Afterward, they lose a lot of strength and cannot repeat the same effort. In this case, doing a second set of the exercise would be counterproductive. However, this characteristic is present in very few people. Scientific research estimates that about 70 percent of athletes do better with multiple sets, and only the remaining 30 percent have muscles that are better adapted for single sets.

The 70 percent group needs to increase the intensity gradually so they can give their maximum to the workout. With a single set per exercise, they feel frustrated because their muscles have not been able to express their power completely. They still have strength left over for another set. In this case, it would be counterproductive to do only one set per muscle. Instead, they should do several sets so the muscle can really work. This is what Burd and colleagues' 2010 research (*PLoS One.* 5(8): e12033. www.plosone.org/article/info:doi%2F10.1371%2Fjournal.pone.0012033) demonstrated. Burd measured the speed of muscle protein synthesis after a workout. Five hours after a workout, anabolic power

- doubled after a single set done until failure and
- tripled after three sets done until failure.

Twenty-nine hours after a workout, anabolism

- doubled with three sets and
- returned to normal after a single set.

Still, these figures require interpretation, because doing three sets instead of one will provoke a stronger catabolic reaction. Therefore, one part of the anabolic response will be wasted in compensating for a greater degradation of muscle proteins. However, the superiority of multiple sets seems well established among the majority of athletes.

8 How many exercises should you do during each workout?

During a workout, you can choose from two training strategies for each muscle group:

1. Choose only a single exercise.
2. Do two or three different exercises.

The choice between these two options is not so difficult if you know the advantages and disadvantages of each strategy.

A Single Exercise: A Good Strategy for Beginners

The Advantages of a Single Exercise

When you first start, it is better to stick with a single exercise: one for the biceps, one for the triceps, and one for the forearms. For each muscle, you should choose the exercise that is best suited for you (we explain how to pick this exercise in step 18).

Later on, you can add another exercise to add intensity to your workout. You can continue adding exercises as you get stronger.

Fortunately, most people love their routines and are happy doing their favorite exercise. This attitude is best for a beginner because constantly repeating the same movement will improve the technique in executing that movement.

Basically, muscles cannot give their best effort on a new exercise. They require an initial phase (called motor learning) to be able to mobilize all their strength. This is why you make great progress on a new exercise as you continue working out. If you are a beginner who is not used to strength training movements, it is difficult to reach the critical threshold necessary for rapid growth. For a beginner, the best technique for increasing intensity is to know that you did 10 curls during your previous workout and so you need to do 11 today, with good form.

If you change your exercises too quickly, your arms will not have enough time to learn to work really hard during the previous exercise. All the time you spend learning a new exercise means less time that you could be gaining muscle mass. Constantly changing exercises when you do not need to will increase these nonproductive learning periods.

The Disadvantages of a Single Exercise

Some people feel the need to do as many arm exercises as possible during a workout. If this is true for you, then you should do it! With only a single exercise, you can quickly grow bored. Motivation and enthusiasm can diminish just like the joy of working out, which is not tenable in the long term for a workout program. Psychological factors (the need for change and renewal) must be taken into consideration.

A Variety of Exercises: An Advanced Strategy

After 3 to 5 sets of the same exercise, if your strength fails and you are getting bored, the best thing to do is

- pick another exercise,
- change muscles, or
- end the workout.

If your enthusiasm and strength are renewed when you do another exercise, then this is the best strategy. But if your strength diminishes greatly during the second exercise, then this is a sign that it would have been better to stay where you were. At this point, it is clear that you should stick to a single exercise.

9 When should you change exercises?

As your muscles grow, you must constantly switch your workout program. Beginners make fast progress, especially when doing the same workout week after week. As long as a routine is producing results, it makes absolute sense to keep it the same. Changing the structure too often creates negative interference, slowing motor learning and preventing a gradual increase in the intensity of the workout.

However, if you notice that you are not progressing over several consecutive workouts, then it is time to change your program. The first variable to adjust in a workout program is the exercises you are doing.

OVERTRAINING: PRIMARILY AN ISSUE OF THE NERVOUS SYSTEM

Eventually you may find that an exercise that was once easy now causes you to feel weak. The first time it happens, this about face will surprise you, but over time, you will get used to it. The reason for this abrupt change is that if you repeat the same exercises in every workout, you end up frying that neuromuscular circuit. In fact, every exercise uses a specific and unique connection between nerves (which order the contraction) and the muscle (which performs the movement). Constantly using the same neuromuscular circuit eventually wears it out because it has had no time to recover.

This local fatigue makes itself known through the loss of good sensations during the exercise in question. This means it is time to use a different circuit by switching exercises.

10 How many repetitions should you do in each set?

DEFINITION: Repetitions are the total number of times you perform a given exercise in a set (see the definition of a set on page 14). A repetition happens in three stages:

1. **Positive phase:** You lift the weight using the strength of your arms.
2. **Static phase:** You hold the contracted position for a few seconds.
3. **Negative phase:** You use the strength of your arms to lower the weight slowly.

You may wonder how many repetitions you should do in a set, but you should know that there is no magic number of repetitions for improving your results. More than repetitions, what really counts is the intensity of the contraction. Altering the number of repetitions is just a way to make progress, not an end in and of itself. Still, you should adjust the number of repetitions to match your goals.

Goal: Increase the Size of Your Arms

In general, you will gain more muscle mass when you perform 6 to 12 repetitions. But if you can do 13 repetitions at a given weight instead of 12, then do it! In the next set, though, you should increase the weight.

Goal: Increase the Strength of Your Arms for Strength Sports

In activities requiring great explosiveness over a short time frame (such as shot put, powerlifting, or bodybuilding), you should do 3 to 8 repetitions.

Goal: Do Cardio Work for Endurance Sports

To develop endurance or enhance cardiovascular health, you should do circuits of at least 20 repetitions.

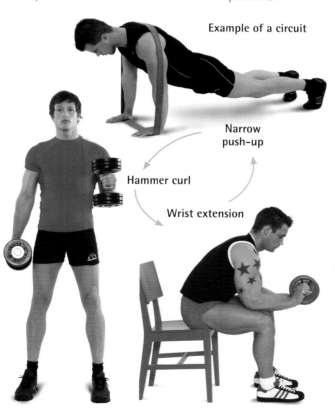

Example of a circuit

Narrow push-up

Hammer curl

Wrist extension

Goal: Increase Explosiveness and Endurance

In activities combining endurance and explosiveness, such as combat sports, rugby, or football, the link between a need for strength and a need for resistance makes the training more complex. You can adapt several kinds of programs to suit your preferences:

1. One workout could consist of a mix of strength work and then cardio work, using the range of repetitions listed previously. The advantage of this strategy is that it better reflects the many muscle qualities required in your sport.
2. Alternatively, one workout could focus on strength work and the next workout could be dedicated to cardio. This way, you will have more rest days between two heavy workouts, which will promote recovery.

PYRAMID DEVELOPMENT

Workouts should be designed like a pyramid. You should start with light weights and a high number of repetitions (25, for example, that can be done easily) to warm up the muscles and joints as well as the cardiorespiratory system. For the second set, increase the weight so that you can easily do 15 repetitions. These two warm-up sets will precondition your arms.

Now the serious work begins: Add resistance to reach the target number of repetitions (based on your goals). But as mentioned earlier, never end a set (except for a warm-up set) just because you reach your target number of repetitions. The more repetitions you can do at a given weight, the more intense the contraction in the arms will be, and the faster you will progress.

As you continue doing sets, gradually increase the resistance (and therefore the difficulty of the exercise). For the very last set of the day, you can either use as heavy a weight as possible or use less weight to really get the blood pumping in the arms. Generally, people prefer one of these two methods. You can also end one workout with a heavy weight and the next workout with a light weight to get the blood pumping.

11 How quickly should you do repetitions?

As you have just seen, a repetition includes three distinct stages. It is best to start by moving the weight rather slowly so that you can learn to master muscle contractions.

The worst thing you can do as a beginner is to move your torso violently while twisting and arching your back to lift the weight. This will create bad habits that will be difficult to break later on. At best, cheating will slow your progress. At worst, you risk injuring yourself! When in doubt, slow down the exercise rather than speed it up.

However, after a few weeks spent learning how to master an exercise, you should change the rhythm of repetitions to suit your goals.

Goal: Increase the Size of Your Arms

To get really well-defined arms, you need to lift the weight using the strength of your muscles and not use any momentum:

– Take 2 to 3 (real) seconds to lift the weight.
– Hold the contraction for 2 seconds and squeeze your muscles as intensely as possible.
– Take 2 seconds to lower the weight.

So a repetition should take 6 to 7 seconds total. Even if you can do more repetitions by going faster, you will be using inertia and not the strength in your arms.

During a set, when you reach fatigue, give yourself a 1- to 2-second pause between repetitions. Let your muscles relax and temporarily regain their strength so that you can do a few more repetitions.

Goal: Increase the Strength of Your Arms for Strength Sports

In this case, the speed of your repetitions is accelerated to add explosiveness:

– Take 1 to 2 seconds to lift the weight (without twisting your body).
– Do not hold the contraction, but immediately lower the weight once you have reached the top of the movement.

– Bring the weight down with control, which means that the descent will take 1 to 2 seconds.
– Between repetitions, take a 3- to 10-second break so that your muscles can rest and recover their strength.

So a repetition should take from 2 to 4 seconds (not counting the rest time between repetitions).

Goal: Do Cardio Work for Endurance Sports

To increase the number of repetitions, use a little bit of muscle inertia, but do not overdo it. Each repetition will be very explosive:

– Take 1 second to lift the weight.
– Do not hold the contraction, but immediately lower the weight once you have reached the top of the movement.
– Lower the weight in 1 second.
– Begin the next repetition immediately.

A repetition should take a total of 2 seconds.

The arms stay permanently contracted. At no time should they be able to rest. When the burn becomes unbearable, give yourself a short break and take a few seconds in the relaxed position. Once the lactic acid has dissipated, begin again until the burn regains intensity. Take another short pause before starting again, and so on.

Goal: Increase Explosiveness and Endurance

The speed of the exercises should match the speed required in your sport. To improve the explosive component, do this work dynamically:

– Take 1 second to lift the weight.
– Do not hold the contraction.
– Lower the weight in 1 second.
– Between repetitions, take a 3- to 10-second break.

To increase the endurance component, do the exercise under continuous tension:

– Take 1 to 2 seconds to lift the weight.
– Do not hold the contracted position.
– Lower the weight in less than 1 second.
– Begin again immediately.

How do you adjust the range of motion in an exercise?

Regarding the range of motion in exercises, there are some commonly held beliefs that need to be challenged.

Dogma: Doing exercises using the full range of motion is the only way to get results. A reduced range of motion happens when you are cheating and will not allow you to make progress.

Reality: A full range of motion seems like a good thing. Unfortunately, over time, it can cause numerous problems. If you straighten your arm too much during biceps exercises, you could cause inflammation or even a tear in the lower part of the tendon (for more information about this, see "Understanding Biceps Pathologies" on page 63). Exaggerating the range of motion in the triceps can cause elbow pain.

In the forearms, the wrists are the weak link because they can be injured when using a full range of motion. It is not easy to build muscle in your arms even when you have no injuries; it becomes impossible if you are weakened by aches and pains. One of the best ways to prevent injury is to adjust the range of motion in each exercise judiciously so that it meets your goals.

Goal: Increase the Size of Your Arms

The range of motion will be the greatest here, but you still need to avoid
- straightening your arms in the lengthened position during biceps exercises,
- straightening your arms too much in the contracted position and bending them too much in the lengthened position during triceps exercises, and
- bending your wrists too much in the lengthened position during forearm exercises.

As you continue doing sets, if you want to increase your weight, you should gradually reduce the range of motion by stretching your arm less at the start of the exercise.

Goal: Increase the Strength of Your Arms for Strength Sports

The range of motion will be slightly smaller here than if you were training to increase the size of your muscles, especially at the beginning of the exercise (lengthened part). Muscles are most vulnerable to injury when you are using heavy weights.

As you continue doing sets, you can shorten the contraction so that you can do a few more repetitions.

Goal: Do Cardio Work for Endurance Sports

It is a good idea to maintain continuous tension as much as possible in your arms, which means that the range of motion will be smaller here. You should neither bend (especially the triceps) nor straighten your arms completely.

Goal: Increase Explosiveness and Endurance

Your range of motion in these exercises should match what is required in your sport.

Still, you must pay attention to extreme stretching, which can cause injuries.

How long should a workout last?

The goal of a good workout is to stimulate your arms as much as possible in the shortest time. Favor a workout's intensity over its length.

The very first criteria that determine the duration of your workout are your schedule and your availability. If you do not have a lot of time, you should know that it is possible to do a complete nonstop arm circuit in less than 10 minutes. However, it is best to have at least 20 minutes. We recommend that you do not spend more

than 40 minutes. If it takes longer than that, it means any of the following:
- You are doing too many exercises.
- You are doing too many sets.
- You are taking too much rest time between sets.

The length of the workout will depend on two things:

1. The volume of work (the number of exercises and the number of sets)
2. The rest time between sets

   This second item is the one you must play around with if you do not have enough time for your workouts.

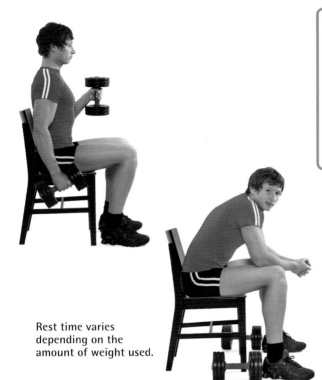

Rest time varies depending on the amount of weight used.

14 How much rest time should you take between sets?

Rest time between sets can range from a few seconds to 2 minutes, depending on the difficulty of the exercise and your goals. You should take

- more rest time for difficult exercises such as pull-ups or narrow-grip bench press,
- less rest time for easier exercises such as concentration curls or kickbacks,
- more rest time when using heavy weights, and
- less rest time when using light weights.

As a general rule, it is time to begin another set when

- your breathing has almost returned to normal, or
- you feel your enthusiasm surpassing your fatigue.

However, before beginning a new set, be sure that you are once again focused on the task at hand. You should

- know how many repetitions to do, and
- remind yourself of your goals.

At first, time yourself so that you stay within the time frame you set. Timing yourself helps you stay in control and prevents you from taking too much rest time. Keeping track of the time will give you more control over the intensity and the total length of your workout.

Your goals will allow you to adjust your rest time more precisely.

Goal: Increase the Size of Your Arms

If you want bigger muscles, there is no point in restricting your rest time. You must give your arms the time they require to recover their strength completely. Using a heavy weight on a muscle that has not sufficiently recovered is counterproductive. However, you should not let everything go and fall asleep during the workout, either!

A good starting point is to take 45 to 60 seconds, depending on your ability to recover. However, you should not rest longer than 2 minutes between sets.

Goal: Increase the Strength of Your Arms for Strength Sports

The heavier the weight you use, the more recovery time you will need. You should avoid working a muscle that has not fully recovered its strength. This explains why you need more rest time for strength work.

A good starting point is to take 1 to 1.5 minutes, depending on the weight you are using. The maximum rest time between sets is 2 minutes.

Goal: Do Cardio Work for Endurance Sports

Rest breaks between sets should be relatively short, no longer than 30 seconds. The goal is to work the muscle again before it has had enough time to recover completely.

One good strategy is to gradually reduce your rest time over several workouts while forcing yourself to maintain (or even increase) the number of repetitions. For example, if you did a workout with 30 seconds of rest between sets, try to replicate the same effort while taking only 25 seconds of rest. If after several sets you cannot continue, then increase the rest time to 30 seconds. During your next workout, try to do even more sets (or even the whole workout) with only 25 seconds of rest.

After an adaptation period, you should ideally be able to train in a circuit. That means combining different arm exercises without any real rest. The only rest you get is while you are transitioning from one exercise to the next. As you continue working out and the circuits get harder and harder to do, you can take 10 seconds' rest between exercises.

Goal: Increase Explosiveness and Endurance

Your rest time should be based on the demands of your sport. For sports that are a combination of endurance and explosiveness, you can use several training methods.

1. One workout can be a mix of strength work with long rest breaks before switching to cardio work with very short rest breaks.
2. Alternatively, one workout could focus on power work with long rest breaks while the following workout would be dedicated to cardio work with short rest breaks.

15 How do you determine the most appropriate weight for each exercise?

More than the number of repetitions or sets, it is the resistance (or weight) that you use in each exercise that determines the effectiveness of your training. It is important to use a weight that is appropriate for your physical abilities as well as your goals.

In the beginning, it may be difficult to figure out the appropriate weight. Some exercises are too easy while others might seem impossible. You may be uncertain, but this adjustment process is not a waste of your time. It helps you develop something called muscle memory. The difficulties in this selection process arise because it is not natural to have to choose the resistance imposed on your arms.

In nature, muscle work adapts to the weight, not the other way around. For example, when you run, your stride automatically adapts to the difficulty of the terrain. In strength training, the logic is reversed. It is as if you were adapting the terrain to the type of stride you wish to have. You have to get your brain and central nervous system accustomed to this paradox. To make the process even more complex, add to the equation the ever-present desire to handle weights that are too heavy in the hope of skipping steps. To find the right resistance in each exercise, start with light resistance and gradually increase it. The following is an explanation of the process. There are three broad weight zones:

- Zone 1 weights seem light and do not require much effort to lift.
- Zone 2 weights allow you both to feel your muscles work and to do the exercise with perfect form.
- Zone 3 weights require you to cheat to lift them, and they do not allow you to feel your muscles working well.

The process for selecting resistance begins with a warm-up. A good warm-up will help you calibrate the level of resistance for your arms. You must always start with a light weight.

You should do your first warm-up set with a weight in the middle of zone 1. The second warm-up set should use a weight from the upper part of zone 1. After that, let your goals determine the amount of weight you use.

Goal: Increase the Size of Your Arms

Do three-quarters of your working sets with weights from zone 2, gradually increasing the weight with each set (pyramid strategy; see box on page 17). This increase should take you from the lower part to the upper part of zone 2.

You can do one last set with a weight from the lower part of zone 3. Handling a weight that is a little too heavy prepares the central nervous system for your next workout. This technique, called future work, is for increasing intensity. Do not abuse it or you could injure yourself!

Goal: Increase the Strength of Your Arms for Strength Sports

After you warm up, do your working sets with a weight from the lower part of zone 3. By gradually increasing the weight in each set (pyramid strategy), you will gradually reach the upper limit of zone 3.

Goal: Do Cardio Work for Endurance Sports

Do your working sets with weights from the upper part of zone 1 and the lower part of zone 2. There is no gradual increase in weight since the goal here is to fight the growing fatigue that happens from doing set after set with little rest time in between.

Goal: Increase Explosiveness and Endurance

Use a weight that reflects the muscular demands necessary for your sport. Two training structures can be used:

1. One workout can be a mix of strength work (with zone 3 weights) followed by cardio work (with weights from upper zone 1 and lower zone 2).
2. Alternatively, one workout could focus solely on power work (in zone 3), and the next workout could be dedicated to cardio (between zones 1 and 2). And of course you will use different weights for each exercise. When you have found the right weight for an exercise, write it down in your workout notebook (see page 26) along with the number of repetitions. The next time you work out, try to do 1 or 2 additional repetitions at the same weight.

WHAT IS THE IDEAL WEIGHT FOR RAPID MUSCLE GROWTH?

In 2009, Kumar and colleagues (*Journal of Applied Physiology*, 106(6): 2026-39) measured the fluctuations in muscle protein synthesis (anabolism) after different strength training workouts. The weight used in the workouts was the same. The only variation was the percentage of maximum strength used for each set. The anabolic response increased by

- 30 percent after a workout with weights that were 20 percent of the maximum,
- 46 percent with weights that were 40 percent of the maximum,
- 100 percent with weights that were 60 percent of the maximum,
- 130 percent with weights that were 75 percent of the maximum, and
- 100 percent with weights that were 90 percent of the maximum.

The anabolic response increases with the weight used. For example, at 75 percent of maximum strength, the increase in the anabolic response equals the combined response of workouts done with weights that were 60 percent plus 20 percent of maximum strength. So, why is the anabolic response not stronger at 90 percent of maximum strength than at 75 percent? The reason is simple: That kind of workout first induces fatigue in the central nervous system, not in the muscles.

Analysis: This information helps you answer a crucial question when creating a workout program: What weight should you use? From this weight, you can automatically determine the number of repetitions that you can do in a given exercise.

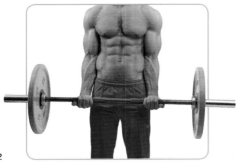
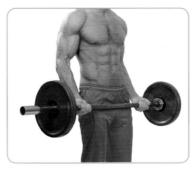

Note: This study also shows that the anabolic response peaks 1 hour after a workout. This is the time when you should eat protein to increase and prolong the growth phase (Moore et al. 2009. *American Journal of Clinical Nutrition* 89(1):161-8).

When should you increase the weight?

The weight that you can use for each exercise is constantly changing. In the best case, your strength increases and you can use heavier and heavier weights. But the natural tendency is to want to jump ahead of this increase in strength and increase your weight too quickly. This means that your form progressively deteriorates during exercises and you feel less and less work happening in your muscles. Finally, you end up losing your motivation because training has become more and more arduous.

Knowing how and when to increase the weight is a critical factor in your progress. To determine if your arms are ready for an increase in resistance, we use two criteria:

1. **The number of repetitions:** When you reach the target number of repetitions (12 for muscle mass, for example), it is time to ask yourself if you need to increase your weight.
2. **Feeling as if the weight is easy to handle:** In reaching the target number, did your form deteriorate? There are generally two scenarios. To increase the weight at the right time, you must absolutely be in the second scenario:

   1. You have artificially reached your target number. There is a natural tendency to cheat more and more in order to convince yourself that you are making progress. In this case, wait one or two workouts, during which time you try to improve the execution of the exercise, before changing the weight.
   2. You feel at ease with a weight that seems too light. In this case, you must increase the weight. The weight increase should be in proportion to how far past the target number of repetitions you went. If you exceeded your goal by one or two repetitions, then you should increase the weight only a small amount.

In general, the smallest increase is 2 or even 4 pounds (about 1 to 2 kg). It is not helpful to increase at a faster rate unless you have really blown by your target number. In this case and this case only, you could do a bigger increase.

Do Not Go Too Fast

The more weight you use (by adding a weight or adding more plates to a machine), the more you risk cheating by using momentum.

Sometimes even a modest increase in weight is enough to cause a considerable deterioration in your form. It is better to increase your weight slightly and often rather than increase by a large amount. A large jump might mean you will need several workouts to rediscover your mind–muscle connection.

If you decide to disregard these warnings so that you can move faster, you will start to lift the weight more with the momentum of your body movement rather than the strength of your arms. You will use more inertia from momentum or twisting your body. You risk hurting yourself, which will slow your progress even further.

Adjust Your Warm-Up

As you get stronger and start using heavy weights in your first set, your warm-up becomes critical. When you are not very strong, your joints, muscles, and tendons do not require a lot of warm-up time since the tension required by the exercise is not high. But as you progress, you should do more warm-up sets, since the tension you are going to put on your muscles is gradually approaching their breaking point.

How much rest time should you take between exercises?

It is not necessary to increase the rest time between two different exercises. Catch your breath using the same amount of time you gave yourself between sets. Increase the time if you feel tired, especially toward the end of a workout. However, you need to move on to the next exercise rather quickly so that your body stays warm, you stay focused, and your workout does not go on forever.

For circuit training, do the exercises with no rest breaks. Ideally, between two circuits, you should limit yourself to a minimal rest break or even no rest at all. After a few circuits, when fatigue sets in, start taking 15 to 30 seconds' rest so that you will be able to do one or two more circuits.

18 How do you select the exercises that will work best for you?

In this book, we have carefully selected the most effective exercises for the arms. However, they might not all work well for you. Indeed, morphologies differ from person to person. There are tall people and short people as well as arms and forearms of various sizes.

A unique morphology should correspond to an individualized choice of exercises. We would be lying if we pretended that every body type could adapt to every exercise. Certain sizes are well suited to some exercises and less so to others. This is the concept of anatomo-morphology, the foundation of the Delavier strength training method.

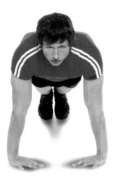 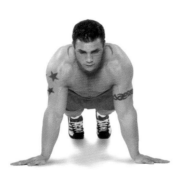

There are two complementary ways to choose your exercises:

1. **By elimination:** Some exercises do not work well with your anatomy. You should eliminate those. Other exercises do not match your goals. These two parameters restrict the possibilities and, therefore, make your choice easier. However, simple elimination should not be your only criterion. Rather, you should find exercises that work well for you.
2. **By selection:** Often, the only way to determine compatibility between your morphology and an exercise is to try that exercise. You will find some exercises that you like right away. But most of the time you will find them a bit strange and they will be hard to do since they recruit muscles that you are not accustomed to using. With time, the novelty will fade and you will feel the contraction in your arms more and more.

Learn to Differentiate Between Exercises

Your choice will be easier once you understand that there are differences between exercises. You should learn to recognize them and use them to your advantage. Every exercise has both advantages and disadvantages. Only by mastering the concept of advantages and disadvantages will you find exercises whose

– advantages most closely match your needs, and
– disadvantages least conflict with your goals.

So we will be particularly attentive to describing the advantages and disadvantages of each exercise presented in the section on exercises (pages 83 to 147). From there, you will have a solid and logical base from which to choose.

A Situation in Constant Evolution

As far as the choice of exercises goes, it is important to realize that things are not set in stone. With time, you will start to enjoy certain exercises that you did not like before. When this happens, your first reaction is to regret that you did not realize it sooner. You might feel that you have wasted time. But this is rarely true, since your mind–muscle connection is constantly changing. A month or two months ago, your arms were perhaps not ready for that exercise. The progress you made means that you can now feel a new exercise very well. So do not have any regrets.

The opposite thing can also happen: You feel less and less from an exercise that you really liked before. This exercise guaranteed rapid progress at first, but now it seems ineffective. This is not just a feeling. It means that it is past the time to remove that exercise from your program. After several weeks of not doing the exercise at all, you can attempt to reintroduce it.

You must constantly adapt to your muscles' development and, most important, be flexible when faced with these changes. This commonsense observation might make you wonder how you can know when it is time to change your training program.

19 When should you change your program?

Some people need to repeat the same training program constantly. This is easy to understand. After all, once you have found something that works, why change it? Other people need things to stay new. It is impossible to know which of these two groups you belong to, and most people probably fall somewhere in between. But your state of mind generally reflects your arms' needs fairly accurately. There are two objective criteria that demonstrate why you need to change your workout routine:

1. **A plateau or regression in strength:** When your rate of progress abruptly stops, it means that something is no longer working. We are not talking about one bad workout, but a tendency that you notice over at least a week. A radical change is required at this time.

2. **Boredom:** When you lose your enthusiasm for working your arms, it means that your program is too monotonous. You need something new! But there are two levels of boredom that you must know how to interpret because they do not require the same kinds of changes to your program. We begin with the kind of boredom that requires the most changes to your program and end with the one that requires only slight alterations in your training program.

   1. Great boredom or even total lack of interest in working your arms: This generally means you have been overtraining. In this case, it is time to take a break or reduce your volume of work. A complete restructuring of your training program will be beneficial.

   2. Lack of interest in an exercise: This means that you have fried the specific neuromuscular circuit for this exercise. You must first change the exercise in question, and you may not need to make any other changes.

Conclusion

There is no set rule for how often you need to change your program. As long as your program is giving you regular results, then why change it? There will always come a time when you will feel it is necessary to make changes. Your arms will tell you by halting their progress. The difference between a beginner and an experienced athlete is the speed with which a person perceives these signals. So be attentive and be sure to keep a notebook (see page 26) so that you can pick up on these clues quickly.

20 Should you take a vacation?

You could certainly train year-round, but this is not necessarily a good strategy for long-term progress. It can be helpful to take a few weeks of vacation every year. In this way, you give your body a chance to rest, and it allows your body to recover mentally and physically. When you want to jump as far as possible, you first need to take a step backward. Similarly, a rest period may help you get past a hurdle that once seemed insurmountable. Even so, there are three disadvantages to taking a vacation:

1. Strength and endurance will decline, but you can quickly get back to your previous level. However, the longer your vacation, the more difficult it is to get everything back.

2. Sometimes a week of vacation turns into weeks, months, and then years. A break followed by a return requires a level of discipline that not everyone has. So, for some people, it is better if they never stop training, because they might never start again.

UNDERSTANDING MUSCLE DECONDITIONING

The central nervous system is the first to respond to training, and it is also the first affected by deconditioning during a rest period. Loss of strength can therefore be rapid. Muscle is more resistant to weakening, so a loss of strength after two or three weeks of vacation does not mean you have lost muscle. So do not worry because your central nervous system will regain its efficiency within a few workouts.

3. Often, a break from strength training means an increase in caloric intake just when the opposite would be better for your body. During a vacation, be mindful of your diet so that you do not gain unwanted weight.

25

Keep a Workout Notebook

It is very important to keep a workout notebook. This lets you quickly see the work you did during your previous arm workout. Your notebook should be as precise as possible without being difficult to maintain. Here is one example:

> Biceps, curls:
> — 15 pounds: 15 reps
> — 20 pounds: 12 reps
> — 25 pounds: 8 reps
> — 30 pounds: 3 reps
> Time: 8 minutes

This way you know which muscle was worked (biceps) with which exercise (curls). Then you find the weight. Normally, people write the weight lifted by a single arm. You could have written 30 pounds which is the total weight represented by the left and right arms. You can decide how you want to track the information. What is important is to stick to the method you have chosen and not write 15 pounds one day and 30 pounds the next time.

Then write the number of repetitions. Here it was 15 on the first set. It is normal to be stronger on one side of the body. In that case, if you do 15 repetitions with the right arm and 14 with the left, write that down so you will know for the next time:

> 15 pounds (R): 15 reps
> (L): 14 reps

To compare two workouts, the workouts should be approximately the same length. End your entry with the total workout time for your biceps so that you can compare future workouts. Time measurement is important because if you rest longer between sets your performance may increase, but it will not necessarily mean you have gained strength. As you lift heavier weights, you will have an annoying tendency to take longer rest breaks. If you note the duration of the workout, you can avoid taking too much time during rest breaks.

Keep all the exercises separate. This way you will know exactly what your goals are for your next workout.

Analyze Your Workouts

After each workout, analyze your performance by asking the following questions:

- What worked well?
- What did not work well?
- Why did it not work well?
- What can I do to make it work better?

Using our previous example, here is a sample analysis that you should do before your next workout:

- Start with a heavier weight because the first set was too easy (you stopped at 15 repetitions but could have done more).
- Continue increasing the weight in the second and third sets.
- In the third set, the muscle was starting to get tired because 4 repetitions instead of 3 were lost for an increase in 5 pounds.
- For the last set, the loss of strength is accentuated with a loss of 5 repetitions for 5 pounds in additional weight. You should have slowed down the rate of increase in weight so that you could do more repetitions (in other words, keep the weight about the same as the previous set). The new workout looks like this:

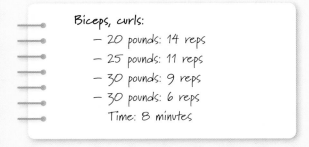

> Biceps, curls:
> — 20 pounds: 14 reps
> — 25 pounds: 11 reps
> — 30 pounds: 9 reps
> — 30 pounds: 6 reps
> Time: 8 minutes

For the next workout, the goal will be to increase the weight by 5 pounds in the last set without losing repetitions. After three workouts, it will be easy to evaluate your progress:

Biceps, curls:
– 15 pounds: 15 reps
– 20 pounds: 12 reps
– 25 pounds: 8 reps
– 30 pounds: 3 reps
Time: 8 minutes

Biceps, curls:
– 20 pounds: 14 reps
– 25 pounds: 11 reps
– 30 pounds: 9 reps
– 30 pounds: 6 reps
Time: 8 minutes

Biceps, curls:
– 20 pounds: 15 reps
– 25 pounds: 12 reps
– 30 pounds: 10 reps
– 35 pounds: 6 reps
Time: 8 minutes

Complete Your Analysis

The pattern that is revealed over a month, rather than what you see from one workout to the next, is what helps you adjust your training program. If the figures increase regularly, then all is well! If the increases slow down, then you must take action by

– changing exercises, or
– taking more rest time between workouts.

In case of a persistent loss of strength, lighten the work load and increase your number of rest days.

Conclusion

Only a well-kept workout notebook can precisely quantify the evolution of your performance over time. Do not trust your memory! Of course you can remember the figures from your previous workout. But how will you remember what you did a month ago? In addition, if you change exercises, how will you remember your past performances when you reintroduce that exercise one or two months down the road? Your workout notebook will be the best witness to your progress as well as an ally in creating future training programs.

Rate of Progress

The very first effects of working your arms are aches and pains. You must view the trauma inflicted on your muscle fibers as a wake-up call that will be more or less brutal depending on your physical condition. To eliminate these aches and pains quickly, you should do another light workout.

After these aches are gone, your strength and endurance will rapidly increase. Basically, your central nervous system adapts to this new environment. It learns to coordinate muscle efforts better while allowing different groups of fibers to work together in harmony.

Even if strength develops more quickly than your muscles do, those muscles will eventually get toned. But as we see every day, it is hard to notice daily progress. So you might feel like you have hit a plateau. And then, one day, you realize that your shirt is tighter and your arms no longer fit well in it.

So long as you are training regularly, your muscles will eventually react. However, it is impossible to determine how quickly your muscles will develop because some people progress more quickly than others. To see your transformation more easily, we recommend that you take photos at least once a month and measure your arm circumference every week.

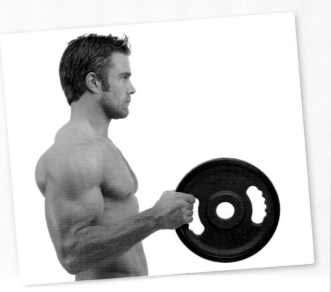

TECHNIQUES FOR INCREASING INTENSITY

The foundation of strength training is overload techniques. You have to overload the muscle in an unusual way to force it to react and grow stronger.

As an example, if you can do 10 pull-ups easily, and you restrict yourself to doing only 10 workout after workout, you will not force your body to adapt. The day you decide to work harder and do 11 or even 12 pull-ups, your muscles will have to provide a tension to which they are not accustomed. They will react to this overload by increasing their strength and size. In the days that follow, it will become easy to do those 11 or 12 pull-ups. So that you continue to progress, you will have to increase the weight.

The easiest overload method is just to do more repetitions with a heavier weight. However, there are other techniques for increasing intensity that will help you progress without adding weight or repetitions.

> ⚠ There are a multitude of techniques for increasing intensity. You should not use all of them at the same time or in every workout. All these techniques have advantages as well as disadvantages. The main thing to remember is that the more intense your workout is, the more time you will need to recover. So you must choose your techniques carefully depending on your goals and your priorities. And as with all good things, do not overdo it!

Volume or Intensity?

Many people confuse the volume of work with its intensity. You must understand that volume of work and intensity are two contradictory terms. As the intensity of your sets increases, it will be harder to do a set. The goal of increasing the intensity is to do the most muscle work possible in the fewest sets possible. On the contrary, the less intense your sets are, the easier it will be for you to do multiple sets. During certain workouts, the emphasis can be on intensity. During other workouts, volume is what counts. But the two must not be used together in the same workout or you will quickly fall victim to overtraining.

Theory of Absolute Strength: A Good Beginning Strategy

The theory of absolute strength says that muscle growth happens when you use weights that are close to your maximum strength. This theory is the basis for strength training, but it is especially intended for beginner and intermediate strength trainers. They need to get stronger to reach the tension necessary for inducing muscle growth.

In your first sets as you climb the pyramid, you have to stop when you are one repetition away from muscle failure so you can avoid fatigue of the nervous system. The more sets you do without forcing yourself to give 100 percent, the higher you can climb on the pyramid while staying relatively fresh. Only when you reach the heaviest sets will you have to give 100 percent.

On the contrary, if you force things as much as possible during the first set, you will get tired very quickly and you will not even get close to your maximum weight.

ADVANTAGES

Absolute strength is better suited for beginners' goals, since beginners need to train with the heaviest weights possible in order to get stronger muscles.

Since they are less tired after the first few sets, they can increase the volume of work (number of sets) that the muscles do.

DISADVANTAGES

Using absolute strength is harder on the joints.

It makes the workout longer, because you are not wearing the muscles out during each set and therefore you have to increase the volume of work.

Inroad Theory: An Advanced Technique

Inroad theory (encroaching on strength) says that to progress, each set must take away as much strength as possible from the muscle. To illustrate this concept, consider a muscle that can lift a maximum of 220 pounds. If you work that muscle with 154 pounds, then at failure, your inroad will be about 66 pounds (220 − 154 = 66 pounds of strength temporarily lost).

When the strength inroad is 66 pounds, this means there is still 154 pounds of strength left in the muscle. If, instead of stopping your set, you take 110 pounds and continue exercising, then at the next failure, you will have an inroad of 110 pounds. You will then be much closer to total muscle fatigue than with the 154 pounds. Many techniques for increasing intensity try to increase the inroad at the end of a set; that is, they try to wear down the strength of the muscle completely (temporarily, of course).

ADVANTAGES

Greater intensity during each set saves time because it reduces the volume of work (number of sets) that the muscles can do.

Greater intensity spares your joints by reducing the strength in your muscles quickly. This obligates you to use lighter weights than you normally would use during subsequent sets.

DISADVANTAGES

Inroad theory is not well suited for beginners' goals since beginners should train with the heaviest weights possible in order to get stronger.

Summary of These Two Theories

Even though we are talking about two techniques for increasing intensity, the theory of absolute strength opposes inroad theory. This difference is especially clear in the different weights that can be used during the final sets.

A reduction in intensity in each set (less inroad) is often perceived as laziness. But it is simply a way to be able to do more sets. The disadvantage of working with very heavy weights (close to your maximum) is the trauma it inflicts on your joints. So you should not use heavy weights in every workout. On the contrary, striving for inroad allows you to stay away from extremely heavy weights, which is better for your joints.

But both of these techniques are traumatic for your muscles in different ways. So you should combine them with workouts that do not put stress on the joints and muscles. This means lighter work in longer sets. So we are left with the following two training cycles.

Beginner Cycle (Beginners do not need as much recovery time as advanced athletes.)

First workout: Very heavy (close to the maximum) with few repetitions.
Second workout for the same muscle: Strive for inroad with heavy weights, but not extremely heavy weights.
Third workout: Very heavy (close to the maximum) with few repetitions.
Fourth workout: Light weights in long sets. Do not strive for a large inroad. This is a recovery workout.
Fifth workout: Repeat the cycle starting with the first day.

Advanced Cycle (Greater recovery time is required.)

First workout: Very heavy (close to the maximum) with few repetitions.
Second workout for the same muscle: Light weights in long sets. Do not strive for a large inroad.
Third workout: Strive for inroad with heavy weights, but not extremely heavy weights.
Fourth workout: Do the recovery workout (second workout).
Fifth workout: Repeat the cycle starting with the first day.

These cycles have the advantage of providing the muscles with the widest possible range of stimulation for growth and strength. For beginners, the emphasis is always on heavy work. Advanced athletes always work with heavy weights too, but they incorporate more intense workouts and active recovery workouts into their routines.

Synchronizing Cycles

There are two ways to do these cycles:

1. **Synchronized cycles:** Work all the arm muscles in the same phase of the cycle, such as heavy day or lighter day.
2. **Unsynchronized cycles:** Work the biceps with heavy weights, strive for a deep inroad for the triceps, and work your forearms with light weights. During the next workout, you rotate these techniques for increasing intensity.

The advantage of the second approach is that it makes workouts easier. With synchronized cycles, heavy or inroad workouts are extremely tiring and light workouts are much easier.

Unsynchronized cycles will let you avoid those truly exhausting workouts. You will work only one or two muscles heavily during a workout instead of all your muscles. The muscles that are lightly worked will have a chance to recover. Your efforts will be more consistent and less extreme.

Here is an example of one workout from an unsynchronized cycle:

Biceps: heavy
Triceps: light
Forearms: inroad

During the next workout, the roles are reversed:

Biceps: inroad
Triceps: heavy
Forearms: light

Should You Train to Muscle Failure?

DEFINITION: We speak of failure when, during a set, the muscle is no longer capable of moving the weight that you have chosen.

Some people prefer to stop during a set one repetition before failure. This strategy does not tire the muscle out as much (less inroad) and so you can do more sets and, ideally, increase the weight more because you have a taller pyramid.

This approach is also appropriate for athletes who do not want to completely tire out their muscles so that they can still train frequently for their sports. There is another strategy where you push to failure on at least your last set, which is a compromise between volume and intensity. You can also push all your sets to failure (striving for a large inroad). The advantage of this technique is that it tires out the muscle more quickly, and so you will not need to do as many sets. The workout is shorter and more intense, and it has a smaller volume

of work. However, the more often you push to failure, the more rest time you will need between workouts for the same muscle.

Beyond Failure

You can also go beyond failure. There are four techniques:

1. Cheat repetitions
2. Forced repetitions
3. Drop sets
4. Rest pause

MEMORY AID

In terms of inroad,
- stopping before failure produces a weak inroad,
- pushing to failure produces a noticeable inroad, and
- going beyond failure produces a serious inroad.

Cheat Repetitions

When you reach failure, it does not mean the muscle has no strength left. It just does not have enough to lift the weight you are using any longer. If you are doing biceps curls with 20 pounds, the first repetitions will seem light since your muscles can lift a much heavier weight. But as you keep doing repetitions, the biceps loses some of its ability to contract because of fatigue. When the biceps no longer has 20 pounds of strength, you can still move your arm, but not as well. Once you have only 19 pounds of strength left, it is impossible to continue the set.

However, by giving the weight some momentum by swinging your torso backward a little, it is possible to finish a repetition that would have been impossible to do with perfect form.

You should cheat *only* at the end of a set. The goal is to make the exercise more difficult by doing more repetitions (beyond what would have been possible without cheating). You must not make it easier by moving the weight with momentum when the muscle does not need it. This is also not about twisting your body all around so that you can lift weights that are heavier than your maximum. Cheating increases your risk of injury, so you must do it carefully and sparingly.

Forced Repetitions

Forced repetitions play the same role as cheat repetitions. They allow you to continue an exercise at a given weight even though the muscle no longer has the ability to do so. For example, during biceps concentration curls, you can use your free arm to support the dumbbell a little bit, bringing the weight to the strength level left in your fatigued biceps. When your muscle has only 19 pounds of strength left and the dumbbell weighs 20 pounds, your free arm will support about 1 pound of that weight. On the next repetition, if your biceps has only 15 pounds of strength, your free arm will support about 5 pounds.

Here we are talking about future work techniques, because the forced repetition shows the muscle the kind of tension it will have to generate in the future to be able to do the additional repetition on its own.

Forced repetitions have two advantages over cheat repetitions:

1. Since your form does not deteriorate, the tension remains on the target muscle.
2. There is a smaller risk of injury.

Ideally, you should work with a partner when doing forced repetitions. But as you have just seen, you can use your free arm if you are working out alone (see more on unilateral training on page 34).

Drop Sets

This technique allows you to continue a set once you have reached failure without having to cheat or do forced repetitions. When doing drop sets, you remove some weight, and this allows you to continue the exercise. In our example of the curls, at failure, you would set down the 20-pound weight, remove 5 pounds, and immediately start the exercise again. When you reach failure again, remove another 5 pounds and continue the set.

There are other ways to do drop sets. In push-ups, for example, when you reach failure, go to your knees. This will make the exercise easier and you can continue.

When you do pull-ups, you can rest one leg (and then both legs) on the floor or on a chair to support some of your body weight. During the narrow-grip bench press, you can use a wider and wider grip, which makes the exercise easier. You can also switch from narrow-grip bench press to push-ups on the floor.

Generally, you should not drop weight more than twice in a set. How much you drop will depend on your inroad. Some people can generate a serious inroad after a single set. They will need to decrease the weight a lot. That is good news in itself, because a serious inroad means that techniques for pushing beyond failure are unnecessary.

However, if you can continue your set by removing only a little bit of weight, this means your inroad is naturally weak. This is generally the case for beginners. Your inroad will increase with experience. In this specific case, it is a good idea to push beyond failure, at least in the last set.

Note: It is important to note that a drop set that reaches a total of 20 repetitions (for example, 10 repetitions to failure; drop weight plus 5 repetitions to failure again; drop more weight plus 5 repetitions to failure again) is very different from a regular set of 20 repetitions. The final number of repetitions is the same in both cases, but it means that dropping weight has allowed you to

- begin the set with a much heavier weight, and
- reach failure three times instead of only once.

Handling heavy weights and pushing your muscles to failure forces your muscles to grow. Drop sets are a very effective way to do this.

Rest Pause

When you reach failure, stop the movement for 10 to 15 seconds to give your muscles a break. After this brief pause, begin your set again. The goal is to do one or two extra repetitions. Rest pauses are often used with very heavy weights. You do the maximum or a double repetition before stopping briefly to catch your breath. Then, try another repetition and so on until the rest pause does not allow you to gather enough strength to do one more repetition.

Beginners who have difficulty with pull-ups, for example, can also use this technique. If you can lift yourself only one or two times, then at failure take a 10- to 20-second break and try again. Quickly, the break will become unnecessary and you will be able to keep doing repetitions.

When you are doing very long sets, it is common to take a rest pause without really being aware of it in order to catch your breath and do even more repetitions.

The rest pause somewhat resembles a stop-and-go (see page 34), but it is different in three ways:

1. The goal is to rest during a set, not increase the difficulty of the exercise.
2. The break from the exercise is longer.
3. If possible, the break does not occur at the beginning of the contraction phase, but rather before the negative phase.

Negatives

Negatives are also called eccentric repetitions. This is the part of the exercise when you lower the weight down. The negative is the opposite of the positive effort, which is lifting the weight. For example, in pull-ups, when you pull yourself toward the bar, your arms and back work positively. When you lower your body, your muscles work negatively because they are only slowing down your descent.

Even though the negative work appears to be easier for a muscle, it is also the most traumatic for the fibers. All the tiny stretches that the muscle does to slow you down cause damage to the muscle cells. The body has to react to this trauma by increasing its strength and developing its volume. This is why scientific research shows that, for a beginner, working negatively is more productive than working positively for gaining muscle mass and strength.

There are four complementary ways to exploit the negative phase of an exercise:

1. Slow the descent of every repetition.

The role of slowing down to increase muscle mass: For beginners who want to increase muscle mass, the negative phase is at least as important as the positive phase. The descent of the weight must therefore be systematically slowed down. However, slowing down the negative phase should be gradual. For example, in a set with 8 repetitions, slow down a little bit on only the first 3 repetitions. Given that it is easier to slow down a weight than to lift it, it would be too easy (and so ineffective) to act too soon on the negative phase. However, as you do more repetitions and your arms become tired, you should slow down the negative phase even more. During the last few repetitions, lower the weight as slowly as possible.

Note: If possible, you should always finish an exercise in the negative rather than the positive phase. For example, when doing push-ups, there is a natural tendency to want to end with your arms straight. But instead, you should stop when you are lying on the floor and you cannot push up any more. The negative movement that brought you to the floor should have been very slow and controlled with all your strength.

⚠️ One mistake to avoid is to hold the weight for 5 seconds at the top of a movement before letting it fall with no control. Slowing down does not mean stopping. Let the weight stretch your muscle by slowing down more and more with every repetition.

The role of slowing down for athletes: When starting the negative phase of an exercise, you can

- let the weight go without trying to hold it, or
- slow down the weight using the strength of your muscles.

A typical example of the first case is weightlifting. In weightlifting there is almost no negative effort. Weightlifters lift the bar. Once they have done the exercise, they let the bar go without trying to slow it down.

But in most sports, there is a negative phase. A typical example is downhill skiing. Contrary to popular belief, skiers' muscles do not work in a static manner. Their thighs are constantly trying to slow down on the ruggedness of the slope. So doing negative work is particularly important for them.

Athletes should therefore analyze the role of negative strength in their sports. The more important it is for their performance, the more they should work on it during strength training.

2. Accentuate resistance during the descent.

The negative strength of a muscle is greater than its positive strength. If you can lift 45 pounds with one arm, you could probably hold back 65 pounds. So an ideal set should contain a negative with more weight than the positive to achieve maximum results. There are three methods of disassociating the negative weight from the positive weight. Intermediate and advanced athletes can use one of them at least every second or third workout:

Use a partner: The easiest way is to work out with a partner who can push on the weight to accentuate the resistance during the return phase of the exercise. Unfortunately, it's not common to work out with a partner. But you can manage without one.

Use your free hand: Working out one side at a time (see page 34) allows you to keep one hand free. This hand can often accentuate the weight on the working arm during the negative phase. For example, during concentration curls for the biceps, you lift the dumbbell normally. When you release the weight, push on the dumbbell so that you add 10 pounds.

Use an elastic band: Special elastic bands for strength training have unique resistance properties. When you pull on a band, it accumulates elastic energy (or strength). When you let go, it will abruptly shorten. In strength training, a band provides an acceleration of the negative phase that no other equipment can provide. This is the main advantage of bands; they progressively accumulate a large amount of tension. This tension will be reproduced abruptly in the negative phase. Your muscles have to work much more intensely to slow down a band than they would to slow down traditional weights. Using a band results in a faster gain in strength, power, and muscle mass than using traditional weights.

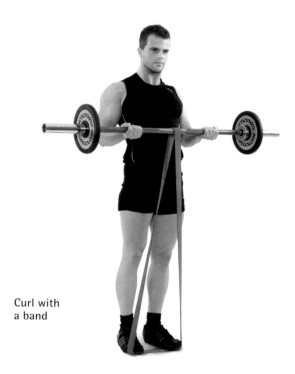

Curl with a band

NOTE

Through the intermediary of muscles (which act like elastic bands), a part of the tension in the band accumulates in the muscle fibers during the negative phase. This strength, coming from the outside, will be used by your muscles to lift the weight. In other words, not only is the negative phase accentuated when using bands, but bands also let the muscles become immediately stronger and lift heavier weights. There is a double benefit that explains the popularity of this training method in strength sports.

3. Use pure negatives.

To be able to give your maximum in the negative, eliminate the positive phase. The exercise consists of just struggling against gravity with the heaviest weight possible. This technique is particularly appropriate when you do not have enough strength to do pull-ups, for example. In this case, you always have enough strength to slow down the descent. The goal is to slow the descent for as long as possible and as many times as possible. The magic of pure negatives is that they allow you to quickly gain enough strength so that you can lift your body all by yourself. In general, two weeks of pure negative training at the pull-up bar will allow a person who was not capable of doing a pull-up to do a pull-up once or twice all by himself.

Another technique is to lift the weight with both arms but to lower it with only one arm. For example, when doing push-ups, lift yourself up normally with both arms. Once your arms are straight, transfer your body weight to one arm and do a pure negative. Be sure that you are at a high enough fitness level before attempting this variation. If you cannot stop yourself, especially at the end, you can do a partial negative. This means lowering 4 to 8 inches (10-20 cm) before going back up using both arms. Alternatively, you can do this negative while your body weight rests on your knees rather than the balls of your feet.

Quickly your increased strength will allow you to go all the way down without any problems.

Many exercises (but unfortunately not all of them) lend themselves to pure negatives. Use this strategy at least once a month.

4. Use postfailure negatives.

You can adopt a slightly different strategy to go beyond failure. For example, do as many push-ups as you can. At failure, use your legs to reposition yourself with your arms extended. From there, lower yourself slowly. Once you are on the floor, get back up using your legs and then repeat for a pure negative. You can use this strategy at the pull-up bar by pushing on the floor or on a chair to get back up into the contracted position.

Stop-and-Go

This technique involves pausing for 1 second between the negative phase of the exercise and the contraction. For example, when doing push-ups, remain lying on the floor for 1 second. Relax your muscles and then activate them, causing the contraction. The goal of this pause is to eliminate the elastic energy that accumulated during the negative phase of the exercise.

The stop-and-go strategy has three practical applications:

1. It is useful in activities that require great initial strength, like throwing a punch. In this case, the arm muscles need to contract as powerfully as possible without being previously stretched. They are relatively weak, yet you are forcing them to be immediately powerful. This is a physical quality that you can develop using the stop-and-go technique.

2. Stop-and-go alters the muscles' recruitment structure. For example, when doing push-ups normally, you might really feel the work in your chest, but not so much in your triceps. By pausing just before the contraction, you might be able to overcome this problem. Many people will feel a different kind of muscle work, which could be oriented more toward the triceps. So, if an exercise is not correctly targeting a muscle, give it a second chance by doing it with the stop-and-go method.

3. Certain fragile joints, like the shoulders, cannot always handle the pressure generated on the tendons at the moment the exercise moves from the eccentric phase to the concentric phase. This transition can be softened with the pause required using the stop-and-go method.

All exercises can be done with the stop-and-go method. This variation will produce benefits with certain movements, but not with all of them. It is up to you to test it out and determine for yourself which exercises work best with this technique.

Burn

When lactic acid accumulates in the muscles during a set, it is called burn. This burning means that it is difficult for the muscle to maintain the intensity of the effort you are demanding. It is a sign of muscle overload.

As with pain, burn is an obstacle to performance. The goal of burn is to turn the obstacle around and make it into a strength. Instead of avoiding burn, you will try to create it because it means there is stimulation that will force the muscle to grow larger. Once you have generated burn, put up with it for as long as possible before quitting. Generally, burn appears after about 12 intense repetitions. So going for burn is something you strive for during light workouts. Continuous tension, supersets, partial repetitions, or drop sets are good ways to test your will when facing burn.

Continuous Tension

One way to increase the difficulty of an exercise without increasing the weight is to maintain continuous tension in the muscle. This means that at no time during the exercise will you let the muscle relax or recover.

For example, while doing the narrow-grip bench press, when you hold your arms extended, your skeleton is supporting the weight instead of your muscles. In this position, your muscles can recover somewhat from the work they have done.

The principle of continuous tension means eliminating that phase where your arms are straight. The whole time you are doing bench press, you keep your arms slightly bent. An intense burn will quickly develop in the triceps because of the intracellular asphyxiation created. In fact, by constantly keeping the muscles under tension, you are blocking the circulation of blood to those muscles. Without oxygen, the muscles produce a lot of waste (acid) as they synthesize their energy.

The same principle applies to the biceps or the forearms: You never straighten your arms during exercises. Ideally, you should use a mix of techniques: continuous tension and a pause. You begin the exercise using continuous tension. When the pain becomes too much for you, take a rest so that some of the lactic acid can leave the muscles. You can then continue the exercise and do a few more repetitions.

Unilateral Training

Most strength training exercises are done bilaterally, that is, by contracting both arms at the same time. Yet this symmetry of movement is not found in everyday gestures, which are mostly unilateral. Indeed, humans are unilateral beings: We most often use only one arm at a time. For example, we do not throw punches with both arms at the same time.

This natural tendency toward unilateralism explains why humans are about 10 percent stronger when working unilaterally.

Concretely, if you can do biceps curls with a maximum of 110 pounds using both arms simultaneously, then unilaterally, the combination of both arms (what you can lift with the right arm and what you can lift with the left arm) will not be 110 pounds, but about 121 pounds.

There is a loss of nerve effectiveness during bilateral work. One way to see this is when you do dumbbell curls. Start the exercise with both arms at the same time. At failure, you can probably get 1 or 2 additional repetitions if you contract only the right biceps while letting the left arm hang straight. This rebound in strength happens because of the increase in nerve effectiveness when contracting only one side at a time.

However, unilateral training is not always easy to do. For example, it is difficult to do the narrow-grip bench press or pull-ups with only one arm at a time. But you can always find unilateral exercises for every muscle. This is a characteristic that we specify for each exercise in part 3 of this book, found on pages 83 to 147.

There are two versions of unilateral training:

Alternating Unilateral Training

In the example of the curls, you contract the right biceps. Only when the right arm returns to its starting position does the left arm begin to work.

The advantage of this alternating technique is that the right arm rests while the left arm works, and then the right arm works again. The disadvantage is that the nerve impulses must constantly shift between the left and the right, which is not ideal. However, certain sports require this crisscross action (for example, boxing or the crawl stroke in swimming). If this is the case in your sport, then this should be a part of your strength program so that your nervous system is well prepared for this specific difficulty. If not, you can pick the second version.

Pure Unilateral Training

In this version, only one side of the body is working. You do an entire set with the right arm, and then you rest a bit before doing a set with the left arm. Again, you take a small rest before returning to the right side for another set. The central nervous system can express its full power in this configuration. The contraction as well as the concentration on the working muscles will be at their maximum. Athletes whose sport requires such work (shot put, for example) should use this technique generously. Pure unilateral training often has the unique advantage of allowing you to do accentuated negatives or forced repetitions with your free hand. The disadvantage of this technique is that it increases your overall workout time, because you are actually doubling the number of sets that you have to do.

Supersets

Supersets involve combining two different exercises together without taking a break.

There are two broad categories of supersets:

Supersets for Antagonistic Muscles

This occurs when you do an exercise for one muscle and then immediately do another exercise for the antagonist muscle. The most popular superset is to combine a biceps exercise with a triceps exercise.

The main advantage of this strategy is that it saves you time. Indeed, it is no longer necessary to rest between sets. The biceps will recover while the triceps is working. The triceps will rest when you work the biceps. In addition to strength, your endurance will improve.

Supersets for the Same Muscle

This occurs when you do two biceps exercises in a row, for example. The goal here is to increase the intensity of the effort. These supersets are similar to drop sets, but they involve changing the exercise. The second exercise uses less weight than the first, which means you can continue the set beyond failure.

There are three kinds of supersets for the same muscle:

1. Classic Superset
This superset includes either two compound exercises or two isolation exercises. The goal is to do these two exercises in a row to go beyond failure. The sophistication of the other two versions of supersets explains why they are more popular than classic supersets.

2. Preexhaustion Superset

Here, the combination of exercises is very particular. You must begin with an isolation exercise followed by a compound exercise. The goal is to preexhaust the target muscle using the isolation exercise. During the compound exercise, the target muscle continues to work, despite fatigue, with the support of other muscle groups.

DEFINITIONS: An isolation exercise is one that affects only one joint and therefore a restricted number of muscles. A compound exercise is one that affects several joints and therefore a large number of muscles.

Here are some examples of preexhaustion supersets:

Biceps:
curl + supinated narrow-grip pull-up

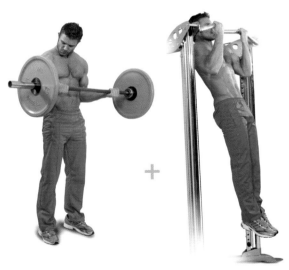

Triceps:
kickback with dumbbells + narrow-grip bench press

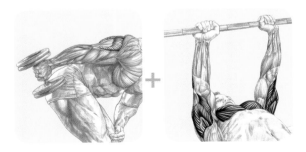

Forearms:
wrist extension + reverse curl

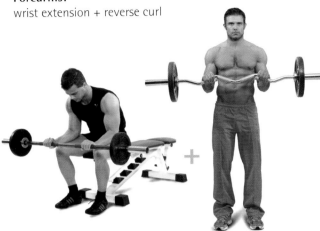

3. Postexhaustion Superset

The logic of postexhaustion is exactly the opposite of preexhaustion. The goal is to work the target muscle to the maximum using a compound exercise. At failure, switch to an easier isolation exercise that lets the target muscle give everything it has left. Postexhaustion supersets are exactly the inverse of those listed for preexhaustion:

Biceps:
supinated narrow-grip pull-up + curl
Triceps:
narrow-grip bench press + kickback with dumbbells
Forearms:
reverse curl + wrist extension

Circuits

Circuits are mostly used by athletes who want to increase functional strength or by people who want to work their muscles and the cardiorespiratory system at the same time. Circuits also make for shorter workouts since there is not much rest time between sets.

In classic strength training, muscle work is segmented rather artificially. You do several sets for the biceps before moving to the triceps. But the body was not made to work that way. In most sports, the muscles work together, not in isolation. However, circuits do not have much of an advantage (except for saving time) if your main goal is to increase muscle mass. Sample circuits, specific to your sport, are described in part 4 of this book, starting on page 166.

How Should You Breathe During a Workout?

Your breathing affects your performance:

- Holding your breath lets your muscles express their full power.
- Muscles are slightly weaker when you exhale.
- Muscles are at their weakest when you inhale.

These physiological reactions are perfectly illustrated in the strategy used by arm wrestling champions. They wait until their opponent inhales, and then they hold their breath and use all their strength to win. In other words, they mobilize all their strength by holding their breath at the same moment their opponent is at his weakest because he is inhaling.

You should use these details to your advantage. In general, strength training books tell you not to hold your breath. This is because those books are written by people who have never worked out intensely. Holding your breath is a natural reflex. Strength, reaction time, precision of movement, and concentration briefly improve when the breath is held. Another advantage of holding your breath is that it tightens the spinal column. In this way, holding your breath protects your back when the spinal column is subjected to great pressure.

Breathing During Heavy Work

The more you work with heavy weights, the more you need to take advantage of holding your breath to optimize your performance. Ideally, you should hold your breath for as short a time as possible. This brief instance of holding your breath should come exactly at the hardest part of the exercise. For example, when you work the biceps by bringing your hands toward your shoulders, the moment when the forearms are parallel to the floor is the hardest. Before and after this angle, the exercise is easier. It would be counterproductive to hold your breath the entire time you are lifting the weight. You just need to do it for a fraction of a second when the forearms reach the parallel position. However, what you must not do is inhale at that particular moment.

Inhale as best you can between repetitions or during the easiest phase of the exercise (lowering the weight). Unlike inhalation, which must be forced, exhalation happens naturally at the moment when muscle pressure is somewhat reduced. But the difficulty in getting enough air during a heavy set explains why that type of work causes shortness of breath.

So correct breathing in strength training is a technique that you will have to learn, and it is much more complex than it seems. It will take time before you completely master it, but it will ultimately prove to be an important part of your progress.

Breathing During Light Endurance Exercise

When the work is light or long, you have to breathe as much as possible to avoid depriving your muscles of oxygen. In this case, it is better to avoid holding your breath, despite the natural tendency to do so. Exhale during the most difficult part of the exercise (lifting the weight) and inhale during the easiest part (lowering the weight).

Breathing While Stretching

When stretching, the breathing logic is reversed. To stretch, you must relax your muscles, but holding your breath during a stretch will make your muscles more rigid. You need to inhale so that your muscles will lose as much tension as possible.

Breathing Between Sets

During rest periods, you must focus on your breathing. Do not hyperventilate and end up dizzy. The ideal scenario is to go to a window for fresh air and breathe calmly.

CLENCH YOUR TEETH TO INCREASE YOUR STRENGTH

Some people say you should relax as much as possible during strength exercises. This relaxation is not natural. All of the muscles are designed to work together, not separately. Therefore, it is not surprising that people are naturally inclined to tense up when exercises get hard. Scientific research has shown that strength increases by about 5 percent when you clench your teeth. It is the same when you clench your fists. What you must not do is tense up so much that it interferes with your breathing.

Warning! Though this tense state is good in strength training, it is not necessarily the case in other sports.

Build Your Arms

The arms are divided into three muscle groups: the biceps, the forearm, and the triceps.

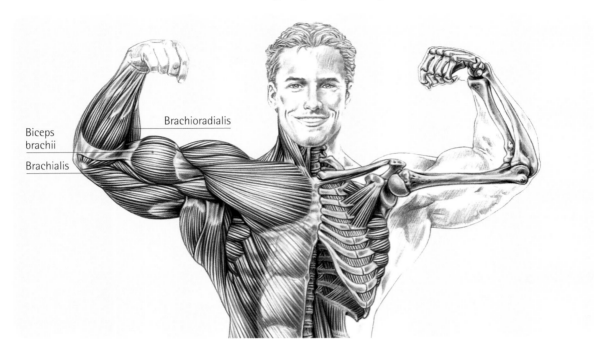

Brachioradialis

Biceps brachii

Brachialis

SECRETS OF BICEPS ANATOMY

🔹 Anatomical Considerations

The biceps has two heads:

1. The long head (outer part), which is the most visible
2. The short head (inner part), which tends to be hidden by the torso

So it is wise to favor the development of the long head if you want to get huge biceps quickly.

🔹 Roles of the Biceps

The arms, and especially the biceps, are the flag bearers of a muscular physique. The biceps is generally the muscle that people want to develop first. Other than this purely aesthetic aspect, the role of the biceps is to bend the forearm and bring the hand toward the shoulder.

It is important to note that outside of its role as an arm flexor, the biceps is the most powerful supinator muscle. Without this muscle, you could not put your spoon in your mouth.

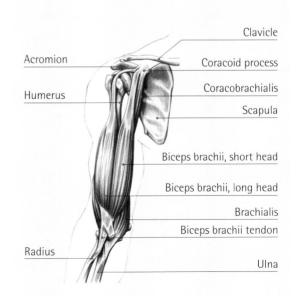

Acromion

Humerus

Radius

Clavicle

Coracoid process

Coracobrachialis

Scapula

Biceps brachii, short head

Biceps brachii, long head

Brachialis

Biceps brachii tendon

Ulna

The Secret to Huge Biceps

To develop massive arms quickly, you must realize that the biceps does not work alone. It is supported by two other muscles:

1. **The brachialis** is located underneath the biceps. It is like a second biceps. The brachialis has the potential to become just as large as the biceps, but this is rarely the case! This is good news because it means there is easy mass for you to gain by specifically working the brachialis. Since the brachialis is not often used in daily life, it is difficult to recruit it in strength exercises. This is why the brachialis is often underdeveloped.

2. **The brachioradialis** is technically more of a forearm muscle. It provides a part of the arm's thickness. Without it, you might have big arms, but they will not be impressive. Even if it adds only half an inch to your arm circumference, the brachioradialis can make your arm look massive.

Only by developing these three muscles in harmony can you get huge biceps.

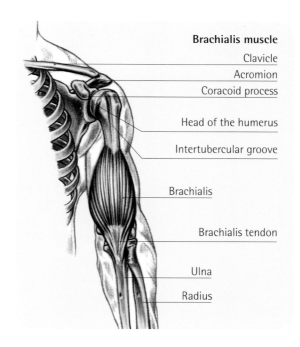

Brachialis muscle
- Clavicle
- Acromion
- Coracoid process
- Head of the humerus
- Intertubercular groove
- Brachialis
- Brachialis tendon
- Ulna
- Radius

Hand Position Affects the Strength of the Biceps

The hand can be placed in three positions:

1. **Neutral position:** The thumb is pointing up. The arm is strongest at bending when the hand is in this position. However, the biceps is not in the ideal position to harness its full power. In this position, the brachioradialis and the brachialis muscles provide most of the arm's strength.

2. **Supination:** The pinky finger is closer to the inside and the thumb toward the outside so that your palm is facing up. This is the best position for working the biceps.

3. **Pronation:** The thumbs are facing each other. The pinky finger is toward the outside. This is the weakest position for bending the arm. Work is primarily done by the brachioradialis muscle while the biceps cannot be of much help.

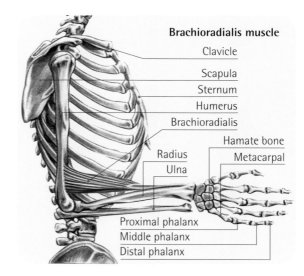

Brachioradialis muscle
- Clavicle
- Scapula
- Sternum
- Humerus
- Brachioradialis
- Hamate bone
- Radius
- Metacarpal
- Ulna
- Proximal phalanx
- Middle phalanx
- Distal phalanx

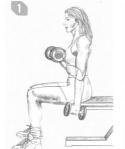
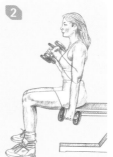
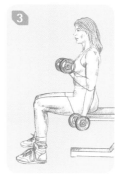

Three ways to do curls with a dumbbell:
1. Mainly works the biceps and brachialis
2. Intense work of the brachioradialis
3. Mainly works the biceps

Hand Position Affects the Strength of the Brachioradialis

1. **Supination:** The fibers of the upper part of the brachioradialis that insert on the humerus are relaxed. The brachioradialis is weakest in this position.
2. **Pronation:** The fibers of the upper part of the brachioradialis are stretched tight. Since tension is not even, the brachioradialis is weakened.
3. **Neutral position:** Tension is even, so the brachioradialis is strongest in this position.

> ⚠ Unlike the biceps and the brachioradialis, your hand position does not affect the strength of the brachialis.

Let's Talk About Size

Impressive arms start around 15.5 inches (40 cm). Really impressive arms measure about 17.5 to 18.5 inches (44-47 cm). Beyond that, arms would really be very huge, but these unusual measurements are very difficult to achieve unless you are already a very large person.

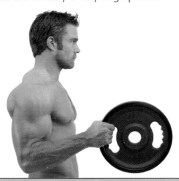

CHARACTERISTICS OF MULTIJOINT MUSCLES

The biceps, the long head of the triceps, and part of the forearms are all multijoint muscles. This means that they attach to two joints at the same time. The brachialis as well as the short head of the triceps are single-joint muscles, so they attach to only one joint. Multijoint muscles are very powerful. They are so strong because their length does not need to change much during an exercise. So unlike single-joint muscles, they can take advantage of the length–tension relationship.

A Muscle's Length–Tension Relationship: The Key to Strength

A muscle's strength is quite unequal along its length. The more stretched (lengthened) a muscle is, the more it loses the ability to generate force. In the same way, the more a muscle is shortened (contracted), the more it loses strength. Between these two extreme positions, the muscle can produce the most tension. This is the muscle's optimal length. This relationship between a muscle's length and its ability to generate force is called the length–tension relationship of the muscle.

The length–tension relationship is not that important for single-joint muscles. In fact, you cannot take advantage of the relationship with single-joint muscles because, when you contract a single-joint muscle, it always gets shorter. However, it is very important to use the length–tension relationship when working multijoint muscles. With these muscles, it is possible to do the following:

- Shorten the muscle at both ends. In this case, the muscles will be relatively weak.
- Shorten the muscle at one end while lengthening the other end. Under these conditions, multijoint muscles can express their full power. In fact, since they are stretched at one end and contracted at the other, they are close to their optimal length, which is the length where they can generate the most force.

This is what happens with the biceps during pull-ups. The biceps shortens where it attaches to the forearm. However, it lengthens where it attaches to the shoulder.

In general, compound exercises exploit this physiological property of multijoint muscles. This is why they are more effective than isolation exercises, which can only shorten the muscle. In fact, muscles develop more easily when they are worked at a length that is close to their optimum.

The length–tension relationship of multijoint muscles is a property that you must absolutely use if you want to quickly gain strength and size. For each muscle you work, you need to determine whether or not it is a multijoint muscle. In addition, for all multijoint muscles, you should know if you are doing a compound exercise (which makes the most of the relationship) or an isolation exercise (which prevents you from taking advantage of the relationship). This is important information that we provide at the beginning of each exercise page.

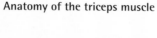

Anatomy of the triceps muscle

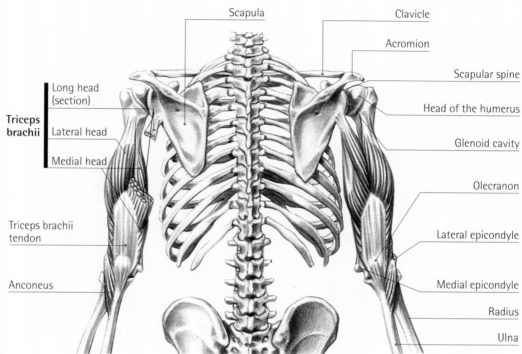

Scapula

Clavicle

Acromion

Scapular spine

Long head (section)

Head of the humerus

Triceps brachii — Lateral head

Glenoid cavity

Medial head

Olecranon

Triceps brachii tendon

Lateral epicondyle

Medial epicondyle

Anconeus

Radius

Ulna

Anatomical Considerations

The triceps has three heads:

1. The lateral head is located on the outside of the arm and is the most visible part.
2. The long head is located on the inner part of the arm and is the only head that is a multijoint muscle.
3. The medial head is largely hidden by the long head.

Roles of the Triceps

1. The triceps allows you to straighten your arm. In this, it is the antagonist muscle to the biceps, brachio-radialis, and brachialis.
2. Working with the latissimus dorsi and the back of the shoulder, the long head brings the arm toward the body. Because of this, it is recruited in all back exercises.

The Secret to Huge Triceps

Ideally, the triceps should be a little bigger than the biceps and brachialis combined. Unfortunately, it is often underdeveloped. But by working it regularly, you can quickly add to your arm circumference.

Of the three heads of the triceps, the lateral head is the most visible, so you need to focus on developing it if you want to have nice arms. If the lateral head is not developed, then your arms will look much smaller.

Aesthetic importance of the lateral head of the triceps

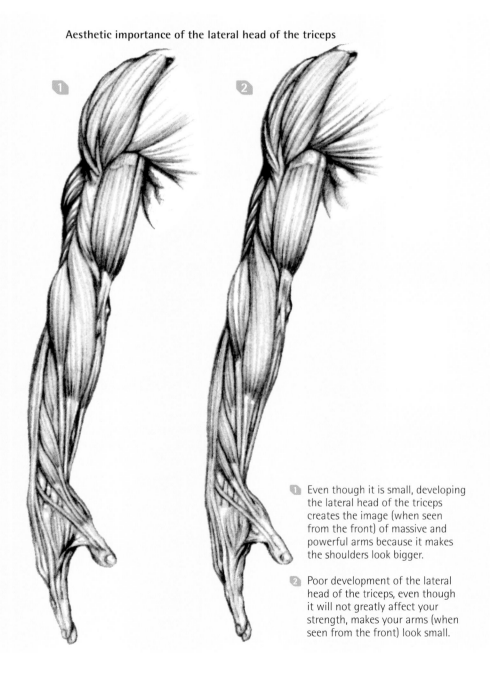

1. Even though it is small, developing the lateral head of the triceps creates the image (when seen from the front) of massive and powerful arms because it makes the shoulders look bigger.

2. Poor development of the lateral head of the triceps, even though it will not greatly affect your strength, makes your arms (when seen from the front) look small.

SECRETS OF FOREARM ANATOMY

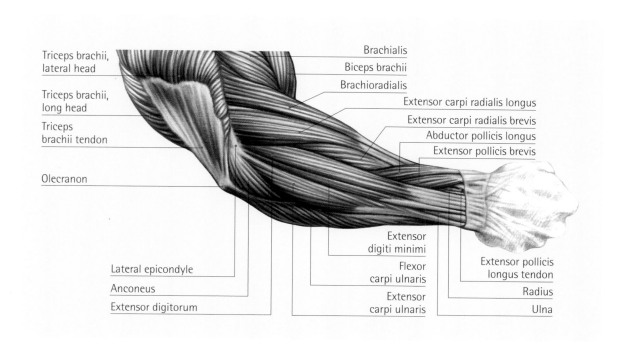

Triceps brachii, lateral head

Triceps brachii, long head

Triceps brachii tendon

Olecranon

Lateral epicondyle

Anconeus

Extensor digitorum

Brachialis

Biceps brachii

Brachioradialis

Extensor carpi radialis longus

Extensor carpi radialis brevis

Abductor pollicis longus

Extensor pollicis brevis

Extensor digiti minimi

Flexor carpi ulnaris

Extensor carpi ulnaris

Extensor pollicis longus tendon

Radius

Ulna

Anatomical Considerations

The muscles in the forearms are numerous and complex, and many of them are multijoint. We are particularly interested in these muscles:

- Brachioradialis
- Wrist flexors
- Wrist extensors

Roles of the Forearms

The muscles in the forearms act in the following ways:

- On the hand by closing, opening, and turning it
- On the wrist by raising and lowering the hand
- On the elbow by raising and lowering the forearm

The forearms participate in almost all arm and torso exercises. Their strength can prove to be a limiting factor in many exercises and numerous sports. If they are weak, then you need to strengthen them.

Practical Observations: The Forearm, a Muscle of Extremes

The forearms are full of paradoxes:

- Some people have enormous forearms even without strength training.
- Other people have modest muscle mass no matter what they do.
- Even with very little muscle mass, some people are capable of extraordinary feats of strength with their hands, such as twisting nails with surprising ease.

The forearms, along with the calves, are the only muscles where such extremes exist side by side. As a general rule, the ease or difficulty you will experience in developing a muscle is closely linked to its length:

- The longer a muscle is (and therefore the shorter its tendons are), the easier it is to develop.
- The shorter a muscle is (and therefore the longer its tendons are), the harder it is to develop.

PART 2

Weak Areas and Pathologies

FOUR OBSTACLES TO DEVELOPING THE BICEPS

You must overcome four problems in order to develop biceps. After reviewing these obstacles, we will explain how to move past them on page 49 ("Strategies for Developing the Biceps").

Small Biceps

This is the main frustration for many people in strength training. Even though you can never have big enough biceps, some people's arms just seem resistant to growth. Visually, small biceps can be dwarfed by large shoulders. The situation is not hopeless. There are innovative strategies, often overlooked, that can help you develop your biceps quickly.

Short Biceps

A biceps muscle is short when it stops very high above the forearm; this is often the reason for poor muscle development. On the contrary, people with very long biceps (that come far down on the forearm) have an easier time developing the muscle.

The only advantage of short biceps is that they have a better peak (the summit of your biceps when contracted). Long biceps have a less pronounced peak.

Unfortunately, you cannot lengthen your biceps. But even though you cannot make your biceps go lower down on your forearm, it is possible to make your forearm climb toward your biceps by developing the brachioradialis (the muscle that joins the biceps and the forearm; see "Secrets of Forearm Anatomy" on page 43).

Imbalance Between the Long and Short Heads

The long and short heads are not always equally developed. You can see this asymmetry when you contract both biceps:

- Seen from the front, a lack of curve and a small peak mean the short head is deficient.
- Seen from the back, a lack of curve means the long head is lacking.

To resolve this problem, you must isolate the work to the head that is lacking.

Small Brachialis

The brachialis is often underdeveloped. So this is easy mass for you to gain. The brachialis muscle's impact on your appearance does not stop there:

- If one arm is bigger than the other, the size difference is often because the brachialis is more developed in one arm than the other.
- Genetics, in large part, determine the form of the biceps, so a large brachialis can improve the peak by pushing the biceps up.

The problem with the brachialis is not that it develops poorly. More often, it suffers from poor motor recruitment. Many people do exercises that are supposed to work the brachialis without the muscle actually working. You must teach the brachialis to contract by doing specific work on motor learning.

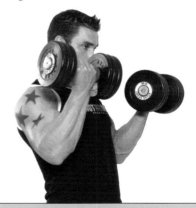

ONE OF MY ARMS IS BIGGER THAN THE OTHER

It is normal for your arms not to be perfectly symmetrical. No one is perfectly balanced, muscularly speaking. So do not worry too much about it. If there is a large difference in size, then specifically working the brachialis will help alleviate the problem.

TWO OBSTACLES TO DEVELOPING THE TRICEPS

You must overcome two classic problems in order to develop the triceps. After explaining them, we show you how to move past them on page 56 ("Strategies for Developing the Triceps").

Small Triceps

The triceps should make up a large part of the arm's muscle mass. Unfortunately, it is often underdeveloped for three reasons:

1. The triceps is a muscle that people may have trouble feeling, and that makes it hard to develop that muscle.
2. The elbow is painful, which makes it hard to work the triceps in the way you should.
3. The triceps is short. It goes from the shoulder (which hides the separation of the deltoid and triceps) and ends very high up on the arm. However, when it is long, the triceps can go very far down on the elbow. In this case, it is much easier to feel and develop it. Unfortunately, you cannot increase the length of your triceps or hide a short triceps muscle (as you can with the biceps). The only solution is to hyper-develop the muscle as much as you can so that the lower part is as visible as possible.

Imbalance Between the Heads

Since there are three heads, an imbalance between them is a classic weak area. Because of recruitment competition between the heads, when the internal part is well developed, the outer part is delayed.

A short outer (lateral) head is often the reason why this rivalry in motor recruitment favors the long head. In this situation, the work of the outer part of the triceps is eclipsed.

The opposite imbalance is rare, but when it does occur, it has two advantages. When the lateral head is very well developed, the following happens:

1. It enlarges your physique. When this head is really muscular, it can be larger than the deltoid. So this muscle, rather than the shoulders, defines your size. If you have narrow shoulders, then you really need to work on the lateral head of your triceps.
2. It improves the separation of the deltoid and triceps by giving the arm an exceptional curve and quality.

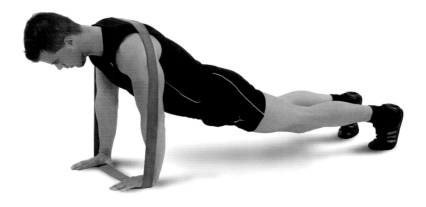

Narrow push-up with an elastic band for greater resistance

FIVE OBSTACLES TO DEVELOPING THE FOREARMS

You must overcome five classic problems in order to develop your forearms. After explaining them, we show you how to overcome them on page 60 ("Strategies for Developing the Forearms").

Forearms Are Too Small

Not so long ago, people purposely chose not to develop the forearms in order to accentuate the appearance of the biceps. This tactic is out of fashion now because body building champions' forearm muscle mass has exploded, especially when it comes to the development of the brachioradialis. It is becoming difficult to no longer consider the forearms as a separate muscle group.

Forearms Are Too Large

The problem with large forearms is that you need a really nice pair of biceps to go along with them. You will not look very good if you have large forearms and small biceps. Furthermore, when the forearms develop rapidly, the biceps have a tendency to lack in strength and appearance. Sometimes, when you have large forearms, you have a difficult time working your biceps effectively. The forearms tend to do all the work, get all the blood flow, and finally lock up, forcing you to stop the set even though your biceps have not worked effectively. Large forearms are not necessarily an obstacle to getting good biceps. You can have good forearms and really great biceps. But when the biceps are not getting bigger, then big forearms will be more of an annoyance than anything else.

Small Brachioradialis

The brachioradialis is often neglected. However, it makes the base of the biceps look thicker and much more impressive. The worst case is when the brachioradialis is extremely short, because then it does not come up on the arm or go down on the forearm. Its absence makes it look like you have squiggles instead of forearms.

By doing specific exercises for the brachioradialis, you can always develop it.

In addition to appearances, a strong brachioradialis muscle will protect the biceps from tearing. If the brachioradialis is underdeveloped, then it can lead to injuries (see Understanding Biceps Pathologies" on page 63).

Imbalances Between Flexor and Extensor Muscles

Working the biceps provides the forearm flexor muscles with a great deal of indirect stimulation. However, the extensor muscles are rarely worked, and this causes an imbalance in development.

Beyond aesthetics, this asymmetry between antagonist muscles is an important factor in the risk of injury. It is possible to decrease or even eliminate some aches and pains in the forearms by balancing your muscle mass through specific extensor exercises (see "Understanding Forearm and Wrist Pathologies" on page 80).

Weak Hands

Even if the flexor muscles are favored in strength training exercises, this may not be enough to strengthen the part of the flexors that specifically provide strength in the fingers. In a gym, you might not be able to grip the bar well, or your performance in sports such as climbing, gymnastics, or windsurfing may suffer. Grip work is imperative!

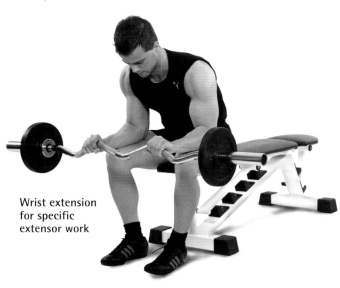

Wrist extension for specific extensor work

2

Strengthening Weak Areas

STRATEGIES FOR DEVELOPING THE BICEPS

Some people can easily develop their biceps while others have arms that seem resistant to growth. However, this is a surmountable problem. Reviewing some of the incorrect notions about this muscle will highlight the obstacles to its growth.

Anatomical Dilemma: You Must Work the Biceps From Every Angle in Order to Develop It

Dogma: Doing biceps work only from multiple angles can develop great arms. This means you need to do as many biceps exercises as possible in every workout.
Reality: There are muscles that have angles, such as the chest or the latissimus dorsi. But the biceps is not really a muscle with angles. Wanting to vary the exercises so that you can work the biceps from many angles means you do not really understand the anatomy of this muscle. Unlike the chest muscles, which have dozens of angles, there are only two angles for the biceps; the others are false angles.

Only Two True Biceps Angles

1. Depending on the elbow position, it is possible to adjust the tension that you place on each of the two heads of the biceps.

The elbow is behind the torso:
The long head primarily does the work.

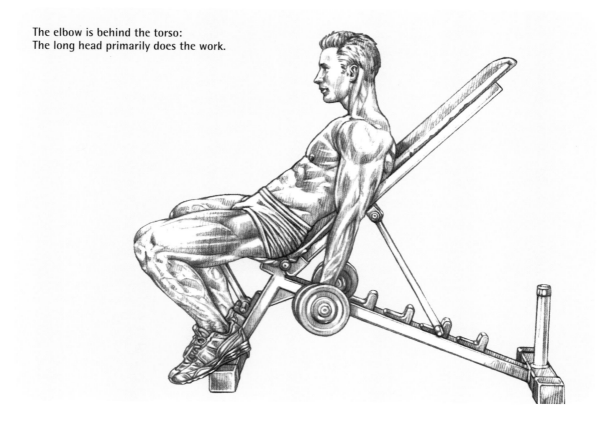

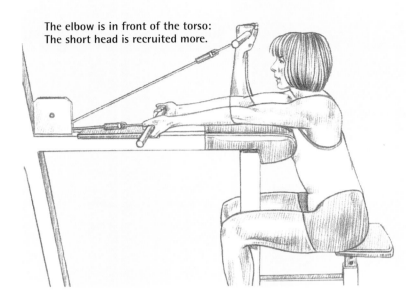

The elbow is in front of the torso: The short head is recruited more.

2. Like other muscles, the biceps are not recruited uniformly across their entire length. Certain zones on the same head will contract more than others. This is called compartmentalization or regionalization. More than the exercise itself, it is the number of repetitions that changes the region of contraction. In humans, type 2 fibers (strength fibers) are found at the edge of a muscle. Type 1 fibers (endurance fibers) are found in the center of the muscle. So if you change the number of repetitions you perform, you can recruit different regions of the muscle.

False Biceps Angles

Depending on your hand position, you can either promote or restrict the contraction of the biceps:

- A supinated grip (pinky fingers facing each other) is the optimal position for the biceps.
- A neutral grip (thumbs facing up) makes the contraction of the biceps uncomfortable. But the brachialis, assisted by the brachioradialis, will compensate for the loss of strength in the biceps.
- A pronated grip (thumbs facing each other) further restricts the contraction of the biceps, and the brachioradialis performs the majority of the work.

The issue is mechanical restriction rather than angles of attack for the biceps. If you are aware of these various phenomena, you will understand better how each exercise affects the arm flexors differently and that it is not really a question of angles.

Hammer curl　　　　　　　Reverse curl

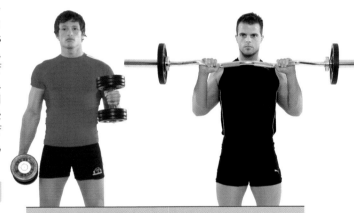

PRACTICAL FOCUS:
HOW TO WIN AN ARM WRESTLING MATCH

The arm is strongest when in a neutral position, which is why you can lift heavier weights when you do hammer curls than when you do classic curls.

In a pronated position, the biceps is weakest, which is why you cannot lift as much weight when you do reverse curls as when you do classic curls. A supinated position falls somewhere in between these two extremes.

There is an infallible technique for beating someone at arm wrestling: Twist your opponent's wrist so that his hand moves from a neutral position to a supinated position. From there, it is easy to beat him because his arm is in a weak position while your neutral position makes you very strong.

Morphological Dilemma: Should You Straighten Your Arms During Curls?

Dogma: If you straighten your arms when doing curls with a bar, you can

- increase your range of motion,
- stretch the muscle more, and
- make the exercise more effective.

Reality: In practice, the fibers that make up the biceps are not really able to bend the arm when the arm is straight and the hand is in a supinated position. The biceps acts by pushing the forearm up to the arm, which puts undesirable tension on its tendon near the elbow. The initiation of arm flexion when the arm is straight is done only in small part by the biceps. The beginning of curls depends more on the combination of brachioradialis and brachialis.

When the arm is straight with a supinated hand, the biceps is in a very vulnerable position. This is why a biceps in a supinated position often tears during deadlifts. At first, the tendons are damaged. If no tearing occurs, there will be inflammation (tendinitis), and it will be difficult to determine its origin. When doing curls or any exercises where the hands are supinated, you should *never* straighten your arms too much, especially when you are lifting heavy weights. Maintain continuous tension.

Choose Your Exercises Judiciously By Analyzing the Anatomical and Morphological Characteristics of Your Arms

To match your morphology to the best exercises for your biceps, you need to analyze two things:

1. The degree of valgus in your elbow
2. The freedom of rotation in your wrist

1. Analyze Your Valgus

No one has perfectly straight arms. To see this for yourself, stand in front of a mirror with bare feet. Straighten your arms with your thumbs as far to the outside as possible. Imagine a straight line that comes from your shoulder and passes through the middle of your elbow. Extend the line toward your hand.

- If it goes through the middle of your hand, then your arm is relatively straight ❶.
- If it goes through the ring finger or pinky or even to the outside of your hand, then you have a very pronounced valgus, which means that your arm is not straight at all ❷.

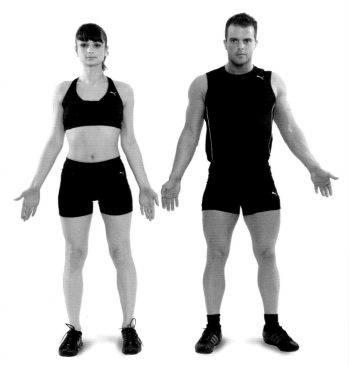

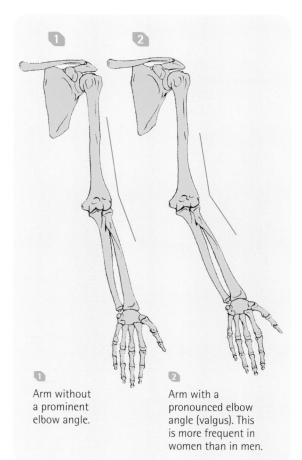

❶ Arm without a prominent elbow angle.

❷ Arm with a pronounced elbow angle (valgus). This is more frequent in women than in men.

The trajectory of movement in the limbs is not the same for every person; it varies depending on your morphology. Elbow valgus is the best illustration of this. See what happens when you do a curl (bend your forearm toward your upper arm as if you were doing a biceps exercise). Keep your thumb as far to the outside as you can, and let your hand come up freely without moving your elbow. If you have straight arms, the hand should come about to your shoulder. If you don't have straight arms, it will fall to the outside, or even far to the outside, of the shoulder.

Anatomical Conflicts

If you have elbow valgus and try to work your biceps using a straight bar, there is an anatomical conflict. The joints naturally want to bring the hand to the outside, but the bar locks the hand into a straight line. Since the bar will not give way, the joints, muscles, or tendons will suffer.

Practically, you will have trouble keeping the bar in your hand, especially in the contracted position. You will have to adjust the bar constantly. This phenomenon is exacerbated in hyperpronators.

2. Analyze the Freedom of Rotation in Your Wrist

The upper part of the radius forms a helix called the ulnar notch. This configuration allows it to articulate with the ulna to bring the hand into a pronated position.

The degree of radial curvature varies among individuals, which explains the large differences in the range of motion in the wrist from one person to another. When you turn your hand, you cannot turn it 180 degrees as you might expect. There are mechanical limitations that reduce your freedom of movement.

These restrictions vary depending on your arm position. When the arm is straight at your side (as when starting curls), the stretch in the biceps limits supination.

With the arm straight and lifted above the head (as at the beginning of parallel-grip pull-ups), the upper part of the tendon on the short head of the biceps strikes the pectoralis major, which limits supination even more. The bigger your muscles are, the smaller the range of motion in your wrist.

Compared to theoretical 180-degree rotation, the average rotation in the wrist is as follows:

- 150 degrees when the arm is bent to 90 degrees. So there is a 30-degree decrease in the range of motion that you gain back in pronation or supination **1**.

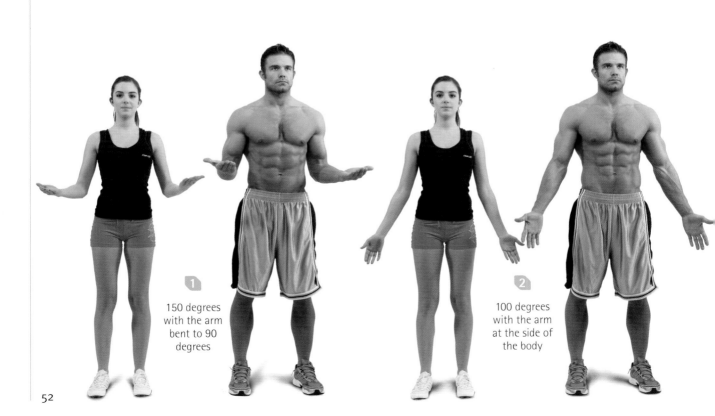

1 150 degrees with the arm bent to 90 degrees

2 100 degrees with the arm at the side of the body

- 100 degrees when the arms are straight at the sides. This 80-degree deficit especially reduces the capacity for supination **2**.
- 90 degrees when the arms are held up in the air. The 90-degree deficit drastically reduces the ability for supination **3**.

It is possible to prove these figures wrong and increase the range of motion in the wrist in the following ways:

- Force the natural rotation of the hand, as happens with heavy weights during curls. Forcing rotation in this way can cause pain in the forearms (see "Understanding Forearm and Wrist Pathologies" on page 80);
- Rotate the shoulder. In this case, the range of motion in the wrist is about 270 degrees. This awkward position no longer involves just the forearm but also the shoulder. In exercises such as pull-ups, repeating heavy exercises will cause trauma not only in the forearms but also in the deltoids.

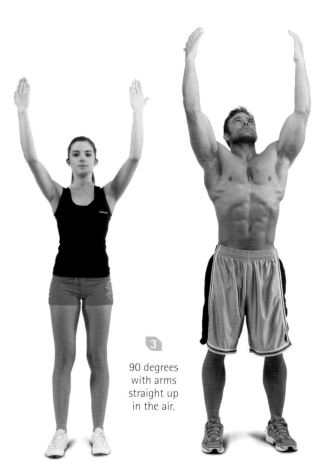

3

90 degrees with arms straight up in the air.

Are You a Hypersupinator or a Hyperpronator?

People can be divided into two broad categories:

Hypersupinators

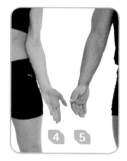

A small degree of curvature of the radius means that a hypersupinator can turn the thumb all the way to the back when the hand is supinated **4**. However, hypersupinators have more trouble turning the thumb to the back when the hand is pronated **6**. This is the decreased range of motion that we described in the pronated position.

Hyperpronators

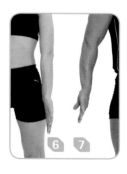

A pronounced curvature of the radius means that when the hand is in a supinated position, a hyperpronator cannot turn the thumb to the back completely **5**. But hyperpronators can easily turn the thumb to the back when the hand is in a pronated position **7**. This is the decreased range of motion that we described in the supinated position.

Conclusion

- Hypersupinators can use a straight bar for curls more easily, especially if their arms are relatively straight (no elbow valgus). Similarly, when using a supinated hand position, it is easier for them to use a narrow grip both for curls with a bar and for pull-ups.
- Hyperpronators will have trouble turning their hands enough to use a straight bar for curls. It will be even worse if they have a large degree of elbow valgus. Hyperpronators also have problems using a narrow grip during curls and pull-ups when the hands are in a supinated position. Hyperpronators should use EZ (twisted) bars or dumbbells, because these tools are better suited for their morphology. Hyperpronators can do reverse curls more easily with a straight bar.

Adapting Exercises to Your Morphology

Struggling to do curls with a straight bar when your anatomy is not suited for it will only cause you pain in your wrists, elbows, forearms, biceps, or shoulders. These issues spread slowly, and sometimes you do not realize where they are coming from. So you attribute them to something other than using a straight bar. By not realizing that you need to give your bent or hyperpronating arm a wide degree of liberty, you can cause yourself pain that seems as if it will never go away.

It is very common for valgus or hyperpronation to be more pronounced in one arm, which underscores the fact that our bodies are not symmetrical. This means that both arms do not follow the same trajectory when they move. In this context, working your biceps with a bar (straight or EZ) could cause crippling injuries.

Practical Applications

A strength trainer who has a slight valgus will get better placement with an EZ bar than with a straight bar. But often, even these twisted bars do not provide enough freedom of movement! For arms that are very bent or not symmetrical, you will have enough freedom to move only if you use dumbbells or a cable in one hand. But sometimes the handle on a pulley can be too straight for a hyperpronator. To avoid twisting your hand too much, you can try attaching the handle so as to mimic the angle provided by an EZ bar.

You will encounter these same problems on machines. The more you straighten your arm, the more the machine pulls your forearm to a place where your hand does not want to go. The machine feels strange. You might think your placement is off or that you are not using the machine correctly. In reality, very few machines can accommodate the trajectory necessary for strength trainers whose forearms have a pronounced hyperpronation. So do not insist on using machines. A good machine is often better than free weights, but unless you have straight arms and flexible hands, this is rarely the case for biceps machines.

Note: If you have problems using a straight bar during biceps exercises, then it will also cause you problems during triceps exercises.

If you take the curvature of your arms as well as the flexibility of your wrists into consideration, you can eliminate many exercises that are poorly suited to your morphology. This will considerably reduce the number of biceps exercises available to you.

Biomechanical Dilemma: Are Curls a Compound Exercise for the Biceps?

Dogma: To build up your biceps, you need to use compound exercises that focus on this muscle. Curls with a bar are the best exercise for the biceps because they are a compound exercise.

Reality: Compound exercises are generally the most effective for gaining muscle and strength. But if this strategy does not give you results, then you need to find something else instead of continuing to struggle with it. This is especially true because classic curls are not a compound exercise. They are typically an isolation exercise for the biceps.

There are three characteristics of a compound exercise:

1. It involves two joints. In curls, only the elbow joint moves.
2. The biceps is a multijoint muscle, which means that it spans two joints: the shoulder and the elbow. In multijoint muscles, compound exercises contract the muscle at one end while simultaneously stretching it at the other end. So the length of the muscle does not vary much during the exercise. During curls, the biceps gets shorter near your elbow, and if you lift your elbow a little bit, it will also get shorter near your shoulder. When a multijoint muscle gets shorter at both ends during an exercise, then it is an isolation exercise.
3. The trajectory of compound exercises basically follows a straight line, while isolation exercises follow the arc of a circle (which is the case with curls).

If Classic Curls Don't Produce the Results You Expect

If classic curls are giving you large biceps, then do not change anything! However, if they are not giving you real results, there is a reason and, therefore, a solution as well. Classic curls do not work the biceps in an optimal way.

To develop a multijoint muscle as quickly as possible, you need to work it at its optimal length. We will look at how the biceps works during pull-ups. The closer you pull the bar toward your neck, the more your biceps shortens near the elbow. But it lengthens near your shoulder. By staying close to its optimal length, the biceps remains strong over the entire range of motion.

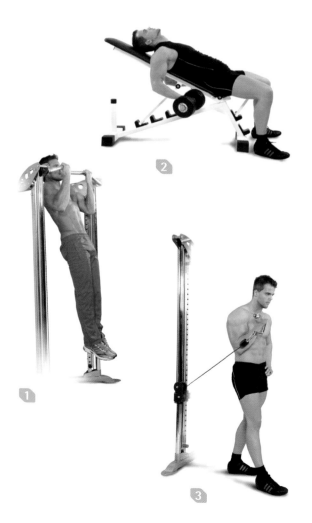

Striving for Optimal Length

If your biceps muscles are not responding to classic exercises, you need to change the length you work them. The goal is to work the biceps close to their optimal length. To alter how you recruit your biceps, use a true compound exercise or put your elbow behind your body.

1. Pull-ups with a supinated grip: This is a true compound exercise that lets you get the most benefit from the length–tension relationship in the biceps.

2. Curls on a nearly flat bench: Occasionally bodybuilders work their biceps on an incline bench, but it is rare for them to use a flat bench. The flatter the bench is, the more your elbow will hang in space, stretching the biceps near the shoulder. This stretch does not happen in any other classic biceps exercise.

   Ideally, you should use an adjustable bench and incline it slightly. This will create a small slope that makes the exercise easier than if you did it on a flat bench. If you place yourself as high as possible on the edge of the bench, the dumbbells will not touch the floor.

   Because of the extreme stretch created by the elbow behind the body, you must start with light weights and do long sets so that you can get your muscle fibers used to the exercise. Using heavier weights can cause inflammation in the tendon of the long head of the biceps near the shoulder, which could cause shoulder pain.

   This is a completely different way of recruiting the biceps, and you will feel more burn in the long head. The long head is the outer part of the biceps, which is the most important part for your appearance. So you should focus on this part first and work the internal part through exercises in which your elbows are in front of your torso (classic curl, concentration curl, and preacher curl using a Scott curl bench).

3. Cable stretch curls with your back to the machine: Normally when you use a cable pulley, you face the machine. But if you turn your back to it, your biceps will automatically get a better stretch, especially if you are working unilaterally. Placing an adjustable pulley at midlevel will give you an even better biceps stretch. To familiarize yourself with this exercise, you should start with a low pulley and raise it a little after each set. The biggest stretch occurs when the pulley is level with your head.

STRATEGIES FOR DEVELOPING THE TRICEPS

To overcome the two classic obstacles with triceps (lack of size and a serious developmental delay in one of the three heads), you should use three different strategies.

Learn to Feel the Triceps

Developmental delays in the triceps are often the result of not feeling the muscle very well. In fact, since you do not use the triceps often in daily life, its innervation lacks sensitivity. If you have difficulty feeling the triceps work, you will have no sense of how well you are contracting the muscle. And, of course, you will not see any results!

As the weeks go by, your mind–muscle connection will gradually increase, but this does not always happen. You should hasten this sensitization by using motor learning techniques.

Repeat So You Can Learn

To teach the nervous system to recruit these stubborn triceps, you must choose the right exercises. Isolation exercises are the most appropriate for accomplishing this task because they reduce the number of active muscles and simplify the movement (see "Exercises for the Triceps" on page 96 and "Advanced Exercises for the Triceps" on page 124).

Once you select these exercises, do the maximum amount of repetitions you can (from 20 to 40) as often as you can. This means that you can do these motor learning exercises every time you work out. Since you are using light weights, the muscle will require only a small amount of recovery time. Do at least 3 sets or even 4 so that 2 or 3 of these sets are working the triceps after it is already tired.

Motor learning exercises can serve as a warm-up before a workout or as a cool-down at the end of a workout. For fast results, do them at the beginning and at the end of a workout. Any configuration is possible.

Manipulate Your Genetics Using Sets of 100 Reps

You can probably guess from the name that a set of 100 means that you do 100 repetitions in a set. This is a motor learning technique that is more extreme than the previous technique and that you use less often (not more than 3 times per week).

Sets of 100 have many advantages for strengthening weak areas:

1. Accelerate the process of sensitizing a muscle to strength exercises.
2. Increase the cardiovascular density of a muscle: Weak spots have trouble getting blood pumping, and there is no better way to increase blood flow to these muscles than by doing sets of 100.
3. Compensate for poor genetics: Often, strong areas are muscles that benefitted from in-depth work done in your youth (such as running, push-ups, and pull-ups). For muscle groups that were inactive up to now and that did not get that kind of conditioning in your youth, you can use sets of 100 to bring them up to speed quickly. After a few weeks using sets of 100, your weak spots will react better to classic training.

Sets of 100 Reps in Practice

Isolation exercises are more appropriate than compound exercises for sets of 100. Machines are also better suited than free weights for sets of 100 because a set of 100 is already hard enough without having to deal with stability issues.

Select a weight that will allow you to do 25 repetitions without having to work too hard. Do your maximum amount of repetitions with this weight (in general, you will get to about 30 or 35). Catch your breath for 5 or 10 seconds so that you can get to 50 repetitions.

Then, depending on your level, you can either reduce the weight a bit or just grit your teeth and keep going. Do 10 more repetitions after 5 seconds of rest and so on until you reach 100. You do not need to do 100 repetitions in all your sets, just for the triceps at the end of a workout.

Evolution: These motor learning techniques will quickly increase the mind–muscle connections in the triceps. Doing this fundamental work will also mean that the heavy training that did not produce results before will now be much more productive.

Strategies for Correcting Imbalances Between the Heads

To get a nicely shaped arm, you need to focus on the lateral head of the triceps first, because it is the most visible. However, to increase strength and power, you need to focus your work on the long head. Unfortunately, nature does not always calibrate the development of a person's triceps with his needs.

The solution for rebalancing your triceps is to reverse the logic of the motor recruitment that led you to your current state. This is easy to do because only the long head of the triceps is a multijoint muscle (see more about this on page 40, "Characteristics of Multijoint Muscles"). To recruit a multijoint muscle optimally, you have to stretch it at one end while contracting it at the other end. This is how the long head of the triceps works during the bench press: As you straighten the arms, it shortens near the elbow and lengthens near the shoulder ❶.

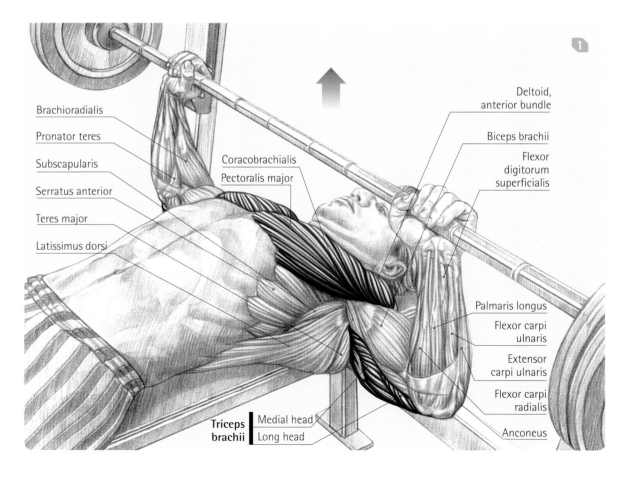

Brachioradialis

Pronator teres

Subscapularis

Serratus anterior

Teres major

Latissimus dorsi

Coracobrachialis

Pectoralis major

Deltoid, anterior bundle

Biceps brachii

Flexor digitorum superficialis

Palmaris longus

Flexor carpi ulnaris

Extensor carpi ulnaris

Flexor carpi radialis

Anconeus

Triceps brachii | Medial head / Long head

You should use a variety of hand and elbow positions in a complementary way to correct imbalances in the triceps. It is up to you to choose the kinds of exercises that best target the head of the triceps that is lacking.

1. Your elbow position affects recruitment of the triceps:

- Using exercises that work the triceps while the arm is at the side of your body will soften the long head and interfere with its recruitment. Mechanically, this will favor the recruitment of the lateral head 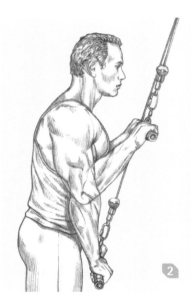 **2** .
- However, when an exercise places the elbow closer to your head, you will stretch the long head and favor its recruitment. Giving the long head priority keeps the lateral head from doing as much work **3** .

2. Your hand position will help you target the part of the triceps that you want to work:

- When your hand is free to move toward the outside during the contraction, the lateral head is recruited more. To do this, you should rotate your wrist gradually to the outside as you contract the muscle. Turn your hand to the outside so that your pinky is up as high as possible. Using the cord on a cable pulley is the best tool for this rotation.
- After that are dumbbells, which allow your wrists to move relatively freely. Various bars (in the form of free weights as well as pulleys and machines) can freeze your hands and prevent you from targeting the lateral head.

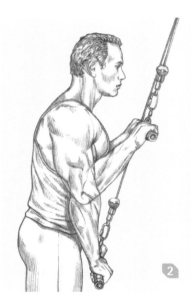

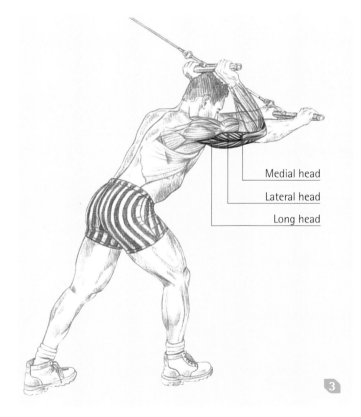

Medial head

Lateral head

Long head

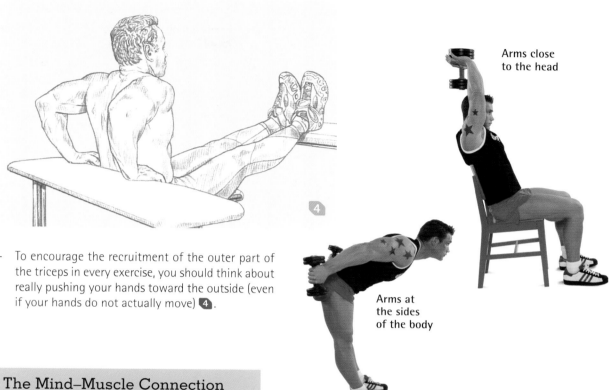

– To encourage the recruitment of the outer part of the triceps in every exercise, you should think about really pushing your hands toward the outside (even if your hands do not actually move) ④.

Arms close to the head

Arms at the sides of the body

The Mind–Muscle Connection

Touching a muscle while you are working it increases the mind–muscle connections and accelerates motor learning. Sometimes you can touch your triceps, especially if you are working unilaterally. For example, when you are doing triceps extensions on a high pulley, your free hand can touch the lateral head to improve the mind–muscle connection.

Is a Fixed or Rotating Schedule Best?

If your triceps development is imbalanced, we recommend that you used a fixed schedule. This means that workout after workout you will choose exercises that primarily focus on the weak head. However, if your triceps development is balanced but lacks size, use a constant rotation of your exercises. If you are an advanced athlete, you should not wait until after you have already fried the neuromuscular circuit to change exercises (see "20 Steps to Developing Your Arm Workout Program" on page 12). By judiciously alternating exercises from one triceps workout to the next, you will allow your nerve networks more recovery time. Here is how to do it:

– **Workout 1:** Pick triceps exercises where the arms are close to your head (focus is the long head).
– **Workout 2:** Accentuate the work of the lateral head by putting your arms at your sides with your elbows as far back as possible.
– **Workout 3:** Repeat the cycle.

The advantage is that the neuromuscular network used by the exercises in workout 1 does not need to be 100 percent recovered for the triceps to be able to function in workout 2. However, it would have been essential for it be fully recovered if you were constantly repeating workout 1 (fixed-schedule approach). A rotating schedule allows you to do triceps workouts more often with only partial nerve recovery.

On the contrary, if you combine different exercises that work all three heads in the same workout, you will need to wait for those neuromuscular circuits to be fully recovered before you work the triceps again. You will have to increase the recovery time between two workouts. With this approach, you will not be able to work your triceps as frequently as you could if you were rotating workouts.

STRATEGIES FOR DEVELOPING THE FOREARMS

When the muscles in the forearms are short (meaning the tendons are long), it is difficult to increase their volume. Unfortunately, you cannot lengthen a muscle because length is determined by genetics.

Paradoxically, having long tendons creates a good lever, which explains why you can have very strong hands even if you have scrawny forearms. This does not mean that your muscles are really strong; it means that you have good leverage.

However, with muscles that are very long and well developed, you can have weak hands. In this case, it does not mean that your muscles are weak; it means that you do not have good leverage.

Get Bigger Forearms

The forearms are generally worked at the end of a workout. Maybe—if you have enough time and energy left over. Often, that is enough. But if you are having problems developing them or if you want massive forearms, then you will need to improve the structure of your workouts by devoting one or two workouts to them each week.

If you have neither the time nor the inclination, you can break up forearm work into smaller chunks. You have many opportunities to work your forearms. We describe all of them so that you have some choices available. You do not have to use all of them. It is up to you to pick the ones that work best for you.

1. Do a few sets for the forearms as a warm-up at the beginning of your biceps workout. In general, this strategy will not negatively affect the biceps workout. However, if you find that it does, then you should skip this strategy.
2. Before working your triceps, some time spent working the forearms will help protect your elbow without tiring out your triceps too much.
3. Between sets for the triceps, you can do some reverse curls to get the blood moving and promote recovery.
4. Because you do not need a lot of equipment to work your forearms (just a dumbbell), you can train at home, using a 5-minute circuit, in addition to your regular workouts.

By working them seriously and regularly when you are not restricted by the training you are doing for other muscles, you can quickly develop powerful forearms.

You can also try some of the suggestions we share for developing good brachioradialis muscles. Those are not a substitute for the ones we just described; rather, they are additional techniques that you can use.

Develop the Brachioradialis

A good brachioradialis muscle has numerous advantages:

- It considerably increases the size of the forearm.
- It fills the gap that might exist between the forearm and a short biceps.
- It protects the biceps from injury.

Even so, this muscle is often neglected.

The very best exercises for developing the brachioradialis are reverse curls and hammer curls. To strengthen the brachioradialis quickly, begin all your biceps workouts with one of these two exercises. If you are focused on rebalancing, you should just start every other workout with reverse curls.

Similarly, as you saw previously, sets of reverse curls can serve as a warm-up before triceps work. You can also alternate triceps sets with light sets of reverse curls to get your blood moving.

There are two cases when a good brachioradialis muscle is essential:

1. If you have short biceps, then you need to develop an exceptional brachioradialis. Because you cannot lengthen your actual biceps muscle, you need the forearm to climb as high as possible toward the biceps. A well-developed brachioradialis will provide that junction between the biceps and the forearm.
2. If the lower part of your biceps tendon seems fragile or is painful, then you should protect it by having an ultrapowerful brachioradialis.

Correct Imbalances in the Forearms

Typically, the flexor muscles in the forearms are used too much while the extensors are often neglected. To correct this imbalance in the forearm, you need to focus on the extensors.

One of the ways to do this is to develop the brachioradialis as just described. You should also do wrist extensions regularly as a warm-up before biceps and triceps work. Do at least 2 or even 3 sets before moving on to reverse curls or hammer curls.

You can also end your arm workouts with these same exercises.

Strengthen Your Grip

Some people naturally have an extraordinary grip. Large hands promote better gripping. But because you cannot make your fingers longer, the only solution is to strengthen the muscles that control your fingers.

If you look closely at the flexor muscles, you see three distinct layers:

1. Superficial layer is responsible for flexing only the wrist and has no effect on the fingers.
2. Middle layer bends the first two phalanges.

3. Deep layer primarily controls flexion of the last phalanx. It is made up of thinner muscles and so is the weakest layer. It is also the layer that is least recruited in strength exercises. When it is recruited, it happens isometrically for the most part, which is not the best way to gain strength and size.

So this layer is the one you need to focus on if you want to increase your grip.

Beyond classic forearm exercises, you should concentrate on grip work using specific exercises that are described on pages 104 and 141 ("Exercises for the Forearms" and "Advanced Exercises for the Forearms").

Evolution: Comparison Between Large Primates' Hands and Humans' Hands

To swing from branch to branch, large primates' hands must be strong and have great endurance. So that they can hang suspended despite their large weight, nature gave them finger flexor muscles that are shorter than those found in humans. So the more a monkey straightens its arm, the more its hand closes, as if it lacked flexibility. Because of this rigidity, a monkey can easily remain hanging from a branch.

The other side of this coin is that a monkey cannot throw an object (such as a rock) forward, which could serve as a defense against predators. Given that the more a monkey straightens its arm as it gets ready to throw, the more its hand closes; the monkey could throw toward the ground only, and without precision.

On the contrary, a human would have a very hard time hanging from a branch for a long period since his hand would eventually open. However, this hand flexibility is what allows him to throw objects forward with precision. So humans were able to become hunters and ensure their survival.

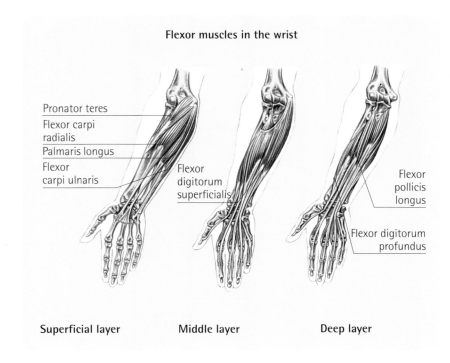

Flexor muscles in the wrist

Pronator teres
Flexor carpi radialis
Palmaris longus
Flexor carpi ulnaris
Flexor digitorum superficialis
Flexor pollicis longus
Flexor digitorum profundus

Superficial layer   **Middle layer**   **Deep layer**

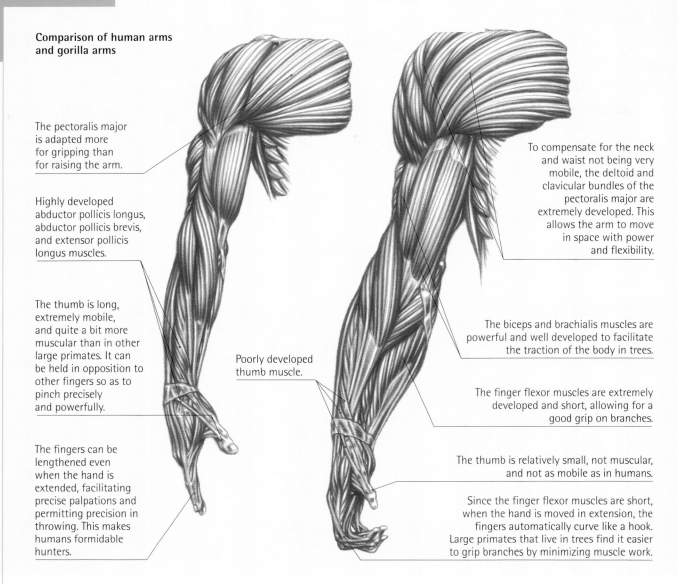

The pectoralis major
is adapted more
for gripping than
for raising the arm.

Highly developed
abductor pollicis longus,
abductor pollicis brevis,
and extensor pollicis
longus muscles.

The thumb is long,
extremely mobile,
and quite a bit more
muscular than in other
large primates. It can
be held in opposition to
other fingers so as to
pinch precisely
and powerfully.

The fingers can be
lengthened even
when the hand is
extended, facilitating
precise palpations and
permitting precision in
throwing. This makes
humans formidable
hunters.

Poorly developed
thumb muscle.

To compensate for the neck
and waist not being very
mobile, the deltoid and
clavicular bundles of the
pectoralis major are
extremely developed. This
allows the arm to move
in space with power
and flexibility.

The biceps and brachialis muscles are
powerful and well developed to facilitate
the traction of the body in trees.

The finger flexor muscles are extremely
developed and short, allowing for a
good grip on branches.

The thumb is relatively small, not muscular,
and not as mobile as in humans.

Since the finger flexor muscles are short,
when the hand is moved in extension, the
fingers automatically curve like a hook.
Large primates that live in trees find it easier
to grip branches by minimizing muscle work.

Prevent Your Forearms From Interfering With Your Biceps Training

People who have strong forearms risk having them freeze up first during biceps exercises. To avoid this problem, you should squeeze your hands as little as possible during the exercise. This is not always easy with free weights, because the bar or the dumbbell could slide out of your hand.

In this case, it is better to work with a pulley. Find the biggest handle you can so that your hand can stay almost open during the exercise. If the handle grip is too thin, you can make it thicker by wrapping a thick sponge around it. At the bottom of the exercise, with semistraight arms, your hands should slightly grasp the handle but not grip it tightly. You should just barely hold the bar without squeezing it. As you contract the muscle, open your hand as much as possible. In this way, all of the work will affect your biceps because your forearm is not recruited as much when the hand is open.

Of course, you should start the exercise with a light weight and do long sets so that you can really focus the work on your biceps. At failure, you can start squeezing your hands because this will give you more strength through the intermediary of your forearms.

But if this interferes too much with the work of the biceps during the following sets, then avoid squeezing your hands at all!

Some machines also allow you to grab the handle with an open hand without the risk of it sliding out. This is an advantage over weights and dumbbells when you need to isolate the work of the biceps.

Preventing Pathologies

UNDERSTANDING BICEPS PATHOLOGIES

There are three broad categories of biceps pathologies. The pain can be debilitating, which is why we focus on prevention. These problems can be prevented only if you understand their cause.

⬤ Causes of Pain in the Biceps

Along with the forearm, the biceps is the location of numerous aches and pains. These injuries delay the development of the arm. Even though people are surprised at how often their biceps hurt, the causes of these pathologies are readily apparent:

- People straighten their arms when using a supinated grip during biceps, back, or chest exercises.
- People with short biceps straighten their arms too much because they want to do what other people are doing, even though their own range of motion is more limited than the average person's range of motion.
- People do not take into account whether or not they have valgus or hyperpronation (see "Strategies for Developing the Biceps" on page 49).
- Even though the biceps is a vulnerable muscle, it is frequently used in torso exercises, which gives it very little time to recover.
- People do not warm up the biceps long enough before working the back, shoulders, or chest.
- There is an imbalance between the development of the flexor and extensor muscles in the forearm, which makes the biceps more vulnerable.
- People with short or poorly developed brachioradialis muscles are much more susceptible to biceps injuries.

1 Vulnerability of the Tendon of the Long Head of the Biceps

The upper part of the tendon of the long head of the biceps requires special attention because it is frequently the location of annoying pain. Pain in the front of the shoulder is often due to inflammation in the long tendon of the biceps. Since the pain occurs doing shoulder or chest work, people often think they are suffering from a shoulder problem. By better understanding the

characteristics of this tendon, you will find it easier to prevent these problems.

The tendon of the long head of the biceps passes through a channel called the intertubercular groove (or bicipital groove). At the end of the groove, it attaches to the humerus and then bends 90 degrees to attach to the shoulder blade. Unlike most other tendons, which are straight, the bone (humerus) rubs on the bicipital tendon when you move your arm.

During exercises such as incline curls, bench press, or dips, the tendon is pressed into the groove, which increases the intensity of the rubbing. It is obvious then how easy it is to damage this tendon.

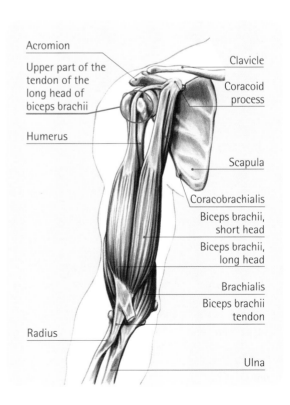

Acromion

Upper part of the tendon of the long head of biceps brachii

Humerus

Radius

Clavicle

Coracoid process

Scapula

Coracobrachialis

Biceps brachii, short head

Biceps brachii, long head

Brachialis

Biceps brachii tendon

Ulna

Brachioradialis muscle showing its helix form

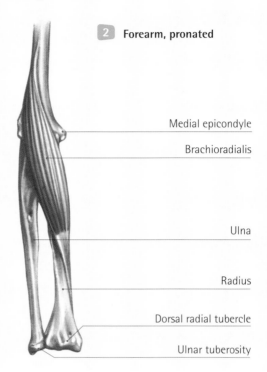

1 Forearm, supinated

- Humeral trochlea
- Humeral capitulum
- Brachioradialis
- Head of the ulna
- Radius
- Ulna
- Radial styloid process

2 Forearm, pronated

- Medial epicondyle
- Brachioradialis
- Ulna
- Radius
- Dorsal radial tubercle
- Ulnar tuberosity

To protect itself from overuse, the part of the tendon in contact with the bone strengthens itself by becoming harder. This explains why the contact surface is fibrocartilaginous. The posterior part, resistant to compression, is necessarily less flexible than the rest of the tendon. By measuring its mechanical properties we can draw some interesting conclusions:

Compared to most tendons, the tendon of the long head is

- three times more resistant to tearing, and
- four times less flexible (so much stiffer).

These values are in line with those of tendons that stabilize bones. In the case of the tendon of the long head, it stabilizes the humerus and therefore the shoulder.

A Fragile Tendon

These mechanical properties suggest the following:

- The tendon was not made to be excessively stretched. The stretch puts its naturally inflexible structure in a bad position and compromises the shoulder's stability. Striving for flexibility in the upper biceps, especially for strength sports, is not wise.
- Structural fragility. Even if the base of this tendon is very solid, the constant rubbing that it suffers will gradually fray the tendon.
- Weak vascularization. This is particularly true in the fibrocartilaginous portion, which is the most used part. This results in a slow regeneration process.
- Rich sensory innervation, which predisposes it to pain.

Conclusion

The vulnerability of the upper part of the tendon of the long head of the biceps can be explained by the 90-degree angle that it forms, the frequent rubbing motion to which it is subjected, and its mixed molecular structure.

A Vestige of Evolution

Why would nature give us such a vulnerable tendon? This structural weakness originates from the sinuous progression taken by this tendon. It was perfectly suited for walking on four limbs, but switching to walking on two legs messed up that system.

Now we must deal with a structural fragility that explains the incidence of spontaneous tears that affect sedentary people over age 40. Of course, the risks are even worse for athletes who move their arms constantly.

Comparison between the upper limb of a chimpanzee (occasionally bipedal) and a man (completely bipedal)

No matter where chimpanzees move in the trees or on the ground, their arms rarely hang down at their sides. The tendon of the long head of the biceps is therefore rarely subjected to friction strains. Unlike a human's tendon, a chimpanzee's tendon rarely has overuse problems.

Because of total bipedalism, human arms continually hang down at the sides of the body. The long head of the biceps is thus subjected to intense rubbing against the humerus. The face of the tendon that touches the bone is therefore covered in cartilage to limit damage from wearing, but this makes the tendon more vulnerable to tension strains.

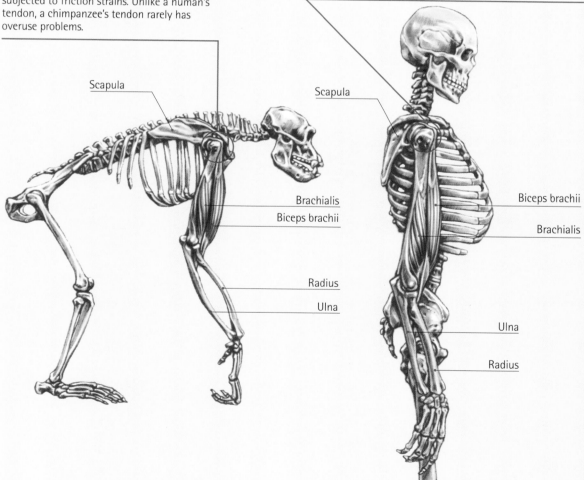

Scapula

Scapula

Brachialis

Biceps brachii

Biceps brachii

Brachialis

Radius

Ulna

Ulna

Radius

Anomaly of the Intertubercular Groove

At birth, the intertubercular groove does not exist. In infancy, the rubbing of the bicipital tendon on the bone will eventually hollow it out. This means that the tendon is typically aligned with the groove.

However, there are four possible anomalies:

1. **A shallow groove:** On average, the bicipital groove is .15 to .24 inches (4 to 6 mm) deep. But in about 20 percent of people, the groove is less than .12 inches (3mm). Because of this shallow depth, the rubbing of the biceps tendon is more intense.

2. **A muscle imbalance:** Doing too many chest and shoulder presses can cause the deltoid to shift slightly forward. The groove is moved back. Instead of passing through the groove, the biceps rubs more against one of the sides, which damages the tendon.

    This bone misalignment is very common in rotator cuff problems, which explains why lesions on the tendon of the long head are found in 90 percent of patients with rotator cuff tears.

3. **Aging:** Over the years or after a sudden fall, a bony protrusion can develop. The bone spurs that are created fill in part of the groove. Their form, which is often shaped like a parrot's beak, ends up fraying the tendon.

4. **A covering acromion:** The form of the acromion varies widely from one person to another. When it is shaped like a parrot's beak, the biceps tendon can strike the acromial arch if you try to lift your arm too close to your head. Gradual wear happens during exercises like triceps extensions with the elbow lifted or shoulder presses. If you cannot completely straighten your arm above your head, it is not a good idea to force it just because other people can do it.

These four potential problems can wear out the biceps tendon prematurely. So athletes' risk of developing tendinitis, or even tearing, in the long head of the biceps is abnormally high.

Humerus, anterior view

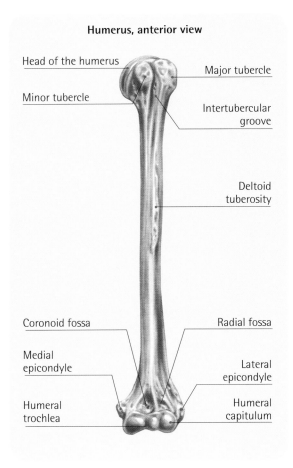

Head of the humerus

Major tubercle

Minor tubercle

Intertubercular groove

Deltoid tuberosity

Coronoid fossa

Radial fossa

Medial epicondyle

Lateral epicondyle

Humeral trochlea

Humeral capitulum

View from below the humerus, showing the depth of the intertubercular (bicipital) groove

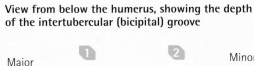

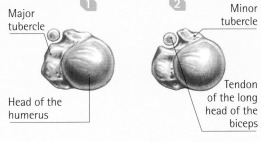

Major tubercle

Minor tubercle

Head of the humerus

Tendon of the long head of the biceps

1. Shallow intertubercular groove: Risk of instability in the tendon of the long head of the biceps.

2. Deep intertubercular groove: The tendon of the long head of the biceps is supported well in the groove.

Recognizing a Problem

The following symptoms indicate a problem with the tendon of the long head:

- Frequent pain in the front of the shoulder after a torso workout
- A clicking in the front of the shoulder when doing arm, shoulder, chest, or back exercises

Touching and palpating the groove (see the illustration of the tendon of the long head on page 63) will cause very characteristic pain. There are three distinct cases:

1. Pain is perfectly localized on the front of the shoulder (the most common case).
2. Pain radiates toward the elbow, hand, and fingers.
3. Pain radiates toward the levator scapulae muscle.

> ⚠ **You must not confuse inflammation in the tendon of the long head of the biceps with true shoulder pain, because the cause of the pain is different in both cases.**

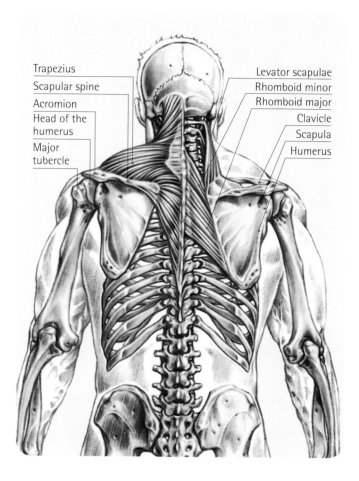

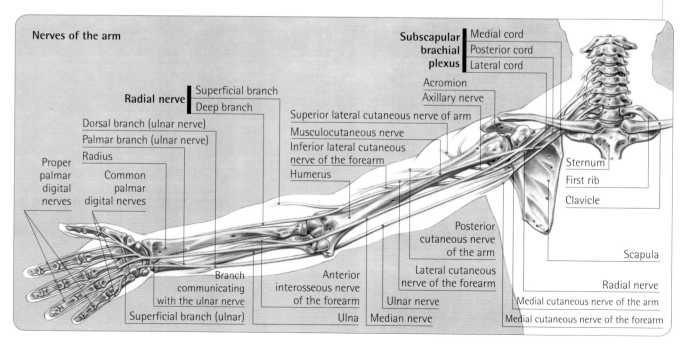

Understanding the Spread of Pain

How can pain from the front of the shoulder spread to the elbow or the arm? To reduce the tension on the tendon of the long head, the upper part of the trapezius and the levator scapulae contract involuntarily. This causes the shoulder blade to rise slightly. This relief comes at the price of tiring out the levator scapulae. Because of the constant spasm, it starts to ache.

Furthermore, since the levator scapulae attaches to the cervical vertebra, its contraction pulls the neck to the side. The cervical curve is changed and compresses the nerves. This feels like pain in the neck, but it can also spread to the arm. Ultimately, it can cause lesions on the nerves, which explains the loss of sensitivity and strength leading to muscle atrophy in the arm.

Prevention Is the Key

To improve mechanical resistance as well as lubrication in the synovial sheath of the bicipital tendon, warm up your biceps well before you work your arms, chest, shoulders, or back.

For your warm-up, do front raises with straight arms using a 2- or 4-pound (1 or 2 kg) weight. Do at least 2 sets of 20 to 30 repetitions.

If you have pain, you must limit the abrasion in the following ways:

– Avoid exercises that press the tendon against the groove (incline curls, decline bench press, or dips, for example).
– Limit the range of stretching in press exercises for the chest and shoulders.
– Do not overdo stretches for the biceps, the front of the shoulders, or the chest. Do not perform these stretches too often or too intensely.

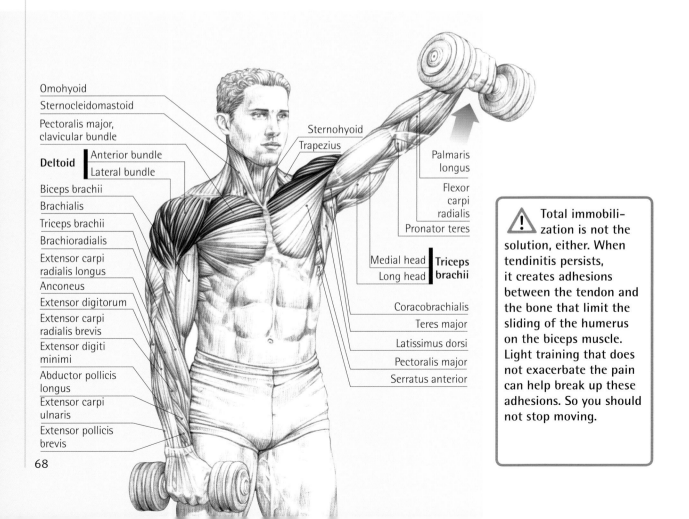

Omohyoid
Sternocleidomastoid
Pectoralis major, clavicular bundle
Deltoid | Anterior bundle
Lateral bundle
Biceps brachii
Brachialis
Triceps brachii
Brachioradialis
Extensor carpi radialis longus
Anconeus
Extensor digitorum
Extensor carpi radialis brevis
Extensor digiti minimi
Abductor pollicis longus
Extensor carpi ulnaris
Extensor pollicis brevis

Sternohyoid
Trapezius
Palmaris longus
Flexor carpi radialis
Pronator teres
Medial head | **Triceps brachii**
Long head |
Coracobrachialis
Teres major
Latissimus dorsi
Pectoralis major
Serratus anterior

⚠ **Total immobilization is not the solution, either. When tendinitis persists, it creates adhesions between the tendon and the bone that limit the sliding of the humerus on the biceps muscle. Light training that does not exacerbate the pain can help break up these adhesions. So you should not stop moving.**

② Three Types of Biceps Tears

There are three kinds of biceps tears that more commonly affect the tendon than the muscle itself:

This is related to the problems just described.

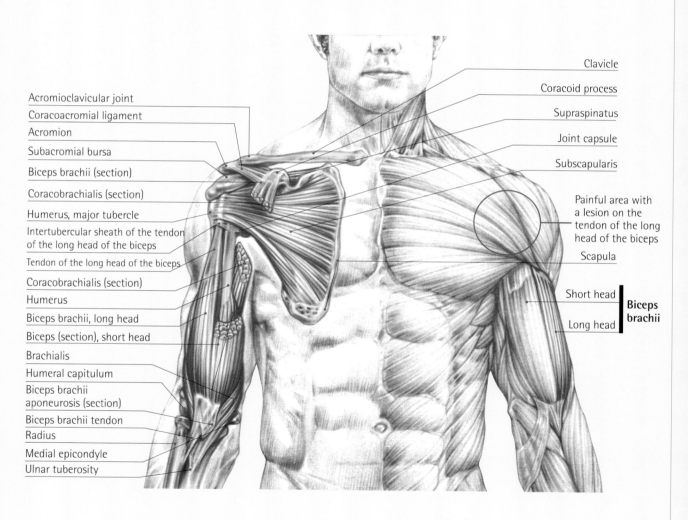

Long head of the biceps brachii, whose tendon is frequently the site of overuse pathologies

Acromioclavicular joint

Coracoacromial ligament

Acromion

Subacromial bursa

Biceps brachii (section)

Coracobrachialis (section)

Humerus, major tubercle

Intertubercular sheath of the tendon of the long head of the biceps

Tendon of the long head of the biceps

Coracobrachialis (section)

Humerus

Biceps brachii, long head

Biceps (section), short head

Brachialis

Humeral capitulum

Biceps brachii aponeurosis (section)

Biceps brachii tendon

Radius

Medial epicondyle

Ulnar tuberosity

Clavicle

Coracoid process

Supraspinatus

Joint capsule

Subscapularis

Painful area with a lesion on the tendon of the long head of the biceps

Scapula

Short head

Long head

Biceps brachii

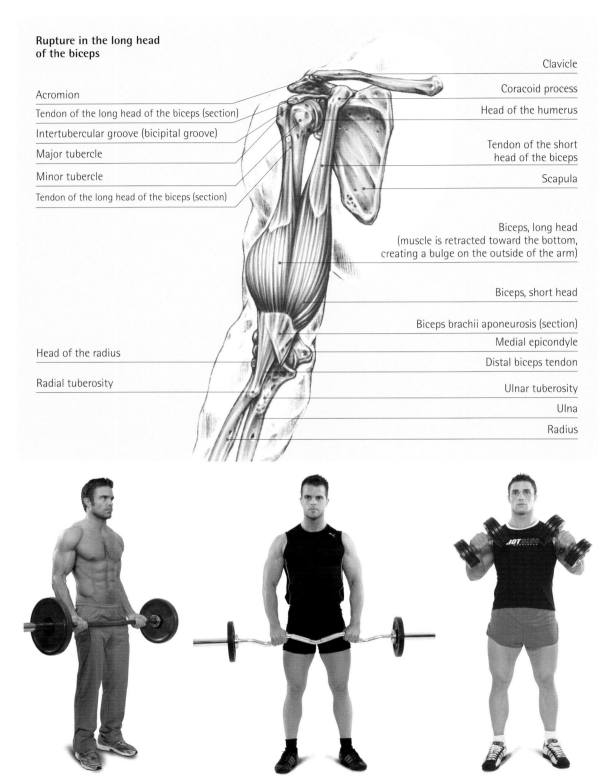

Rupture in the long head of the biceps

Acromion

Tendon of the long head of the biceps (section)

Intertubercular groove (bicipital groove)

Major tubercle

Minor tubercle

Tendon of the long head of the biceps (section)

Head of the radius

Radial tuberosity

Clavicle

Coracoid process

Head of the humerus

Tendon of the short head of the biceps

Scapula

Biceps, long head
(muscle is retracted toward the bottom, creating a bulge on the outside of the arm)

Biceps, short head

Biceps brachii aponeurosis (section)

Medial epicondyle

Distal biceps tendon

Ulnar tuberosity

Ulna

Radius

To prevent biceps injuries, use a straight bar, an EZ bar, or dumbbells that are suitable for your body type and for the exercises you are doing.

Tears in the Lower Part of the Biceps

This injury happens frequently when lifting a weight with straight or slightly bent arms using a supinated grip. This is the case for deadlifts, curls, and pull-ups.

Tear in the biceps brachii

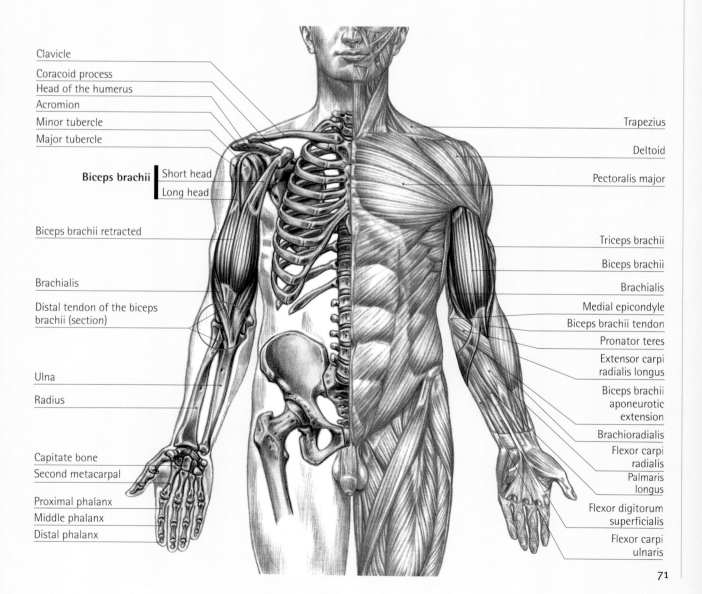

Clavicle

Coracoid process

Head of the humerus

Acromion

Minor tubercle

Major tubercle

Biceps brachii | Short head
| Long head

Biceps brachii retracted

Brachialis

Distal tendon of the biceps brachii (section)

Ulna

Radius

Capitate bone

Second metacarpal

Proximal phalanx

Middle phalanx

Distal phalanx

Trapezius

Deltoid

Pectoralis major

Triceps brachii

Biceps brachii

Brachialis

Medial epicondyle

Biceps brachii tendon

Pronator teres

Extensor carpi radialis longus

Biceps brachii aponeurotic extension

Brachioradialis

Flexor carpi radialis

Palmaris longus

Flexor digitorum superficialis

Flexor carpi ulnaris

71

Tear in the tendon of the short head of the biceps

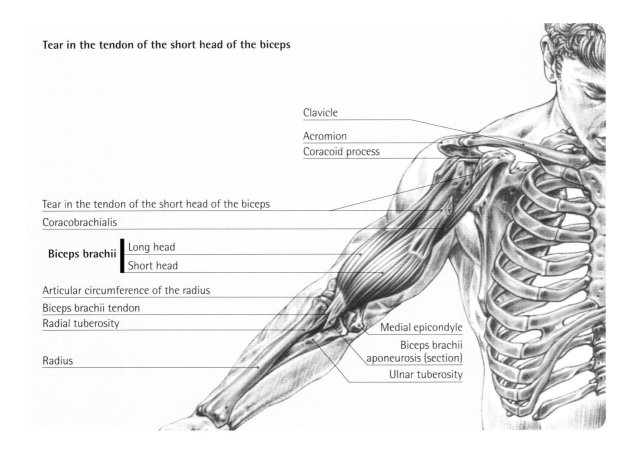

Clavicle
Acromion
Coracoid process

Tear in the tendon of the short head of the biceps
Coracobrachialis

Biceps brachii | Long head
| Short head

Articular circumference of the radius
Biceps brachii tendon
Radial tuberosity

Radius

Medial epicondyle
Biceps brachii aponeurosis (section)
Ulnar tuberosity

Tears in the Upper Part of the Short Head of the Biceps

This kind of tear happens more rarely; it is caused by two kinds of movements:

– **Tears during strength exercises:** This is the case for upright rows, and these are only partial tears. As you lift the bar and bend your arm with the elbow to the outside, the lower part of your biceps contracts and the upper part of the short head stretches. This stretch can cause a tear. This often happens in strength sports such as Atlas stone lifting or, more commonly in daily life, when carrying a large box in front of your body.

– **Pull-ups with a parallel grip on a straight bar:** In this position, the tendon of the short head limits the forearm's ability to supinate. By forcibly twisting your wrist to grab a straight bar, you increase the tension placed on the tendon of the short head of the biceps, especially if you straighten your arms at the bottom of the exercise.

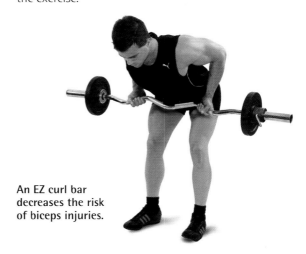

An EZ curl bar decreases the risk of biceps injuries.

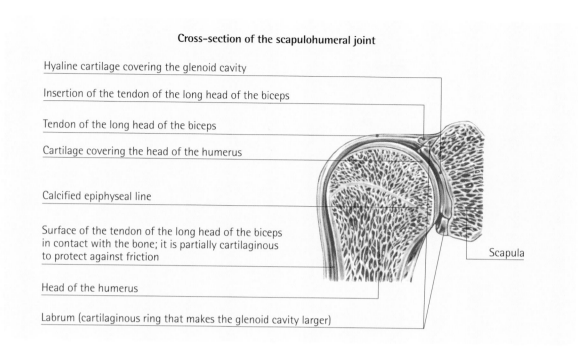

Cross-section of the scapulohumeral joint

Hyaline cartilage covering the glenoid cavity

Insertion of the tendon of the long head of the biceps

Tendon of the long head of the biceps

Cartilage covering the head of the humerus

Calcified epiphyseal line

Surface of the tendon of the long head of the biceps in contact with the bone; it is partially cartilaginous to protect against friction

Head of the humerus

Labrum (cartilaginous ring that makes the glenoid cavity larger)

Scapula

3 Focus on Problems With the Labrum

The labrum is a cartilaginous ring that stabilizes the head of the humerus in the glenoid cavity by increasing the depth of this cavity by 50 percent. The result is that the arm stays in place better in the shoulder joint.

In this, the labrum acts similarly to a rubber washer that ensures the seal between two pipes. But, like all washers, the labrum can deteriorate. When this happens, the humerus starts to float in the glenoid cavity, destabilizing the shoulder and causing pain.

Despite its passive role, the labrum undergoes numerous traumas in athletes.

Understanding Tears in the Labrum

Half of the upper part of the tendon of the long head of the biceps attaches to the labrum. If you pull excessively on this tendon, it can pull the labrum with it and tear it. This is a very common injury for athletes who do shot put. The abrupt forward projection of the arm pulls the humerus out of the glenoid cavity. If the stretch is too pronounced, a space is created that pulls excessively on the tendon of the long head.

The tendon can resist, but at the price of a likely laceration of the labrum. A lesion in the labrobicipital complex forms. This is the infamous SLAP (superior labrum anterior and posterior) tear.

Tear in the glenoid labrum

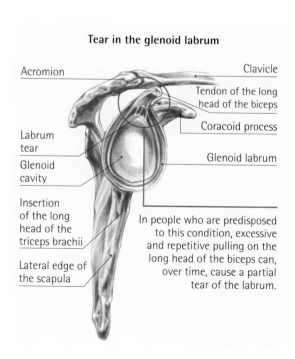

Acromion

Clavicle

Tendon of the long head of the biceps

Coracoid process

Labrum tear

Glenoid labrum

Glenoid cavity

Insertion of the long head of the triceps brachii

Lateral edge of the scapula

In people who are predisposed to this condition, excessive and repetitive pulling on the long head of the biceps can, over time, cause a partial tear of the labrum.

There is another type of problem that happens in certain strength exercises, such as in pull-ups. At the bottom of the exercise, while the arms are straight, if you make an abrupt movement to come back up, the shoulder ligaments must absorb the shock. This shock stretches the ligaments while they are not flexible. Any pulling on the shoulder ligaments can potentially tear the labrum, because some of those ligaments are directly attached to it.

In strength training, there is a phenomenon of overuse caused by frequently doing arm exercises with heavy weights. The shoulder becomes loose, which can become painful.

In contact sports, a collision can dislocate the shoulder and damage the labrum.

Preventing Tears in the Labrum

Once the labrum is damaged, it cannot heal on its own. Even with surgery, there is little chance of a complete recovery. So you should do everything possible to prevent this kind of injury:

1. If you do shot put, you should not stretch the upper part of your biceps too much to avoid dislocating the shoulder.
2. Handle heavy weights with great care during chest or shoulder presses.
3. When doing pull-ups on a straight bar, do not jerk your shoulder. Though it may allow you to use heavier weights, you will eventually pay a heavy price for it.
4. Warm up and strengthen your rotator cuff muscles to anchor your humerus firmly in the glenoid cavity.
5. When you stretch, moderate the intensity of biceps and shoulder stretches.

Two classic injuries to the long head of the biceps

 Overuse and section of the long head of the biceps

2 Tear in the glenoid labrum where the tendon of the long head of the biceps attaches

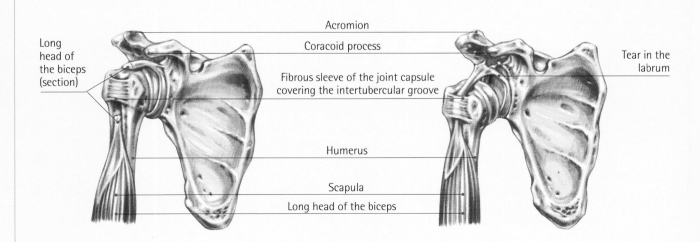

Long head of the biceps (section)

Acromion

Coracoid process

Fibrous sleeve of the joint capsule covering the intertubercular groove

Humerus

Scapula

Long head of the biceps

Tear in the labrum

UNDERSTANDING TRICEPS AND ELBOW PATHOLOGIES

There are two classic problems that affect the triceps: elbow pain and muscle tears.

NOT DESIGNED FOR STRENGTH TRAINING

The triceps muscle was made to throw light objects in an explosive manner as when hunting (that is, using a stick or a small stone). Repeatedly throwing objects that weigh more than 6 pounds (~3 kg) will eventually result in a huge increase in the risk of elbow degeneration.

Unlike the biceps, which is capable of pulling the body's weight, the triceps was not made to generate intense contractions. The elbows were not meant to stretch the arm when facing strong resistance, as required in strength training. So, working out with weights can easily lead to premature overuse of the elbow and ultimately to elbow pain.

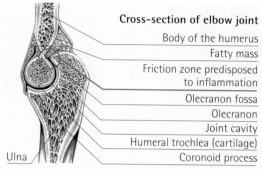

Cross-section of elbow joint
- Body of the humerus
- Fatty mass
- Friction zone predisposed to inflammation
- Olecranon fossa
- Olecranon
- Joint cavity
- Humeral trochlea (cartilage)
- Coronoid process
- Ulna

With repeated extension of the forearm, the olecranon strikes the olecranon fossa of the humerus. Thus the joint suffers microtraumas that can eventually create painful inflammation in the dorsal side of the elbow.

1 Understanding Elbow Pain

Even though the triceps is less vulnerable than the biceps, there can still be numerous problems near the elbow that could debilitate an athlete.

The elbow is a very exposed joint. In addition to triceps work, chest and shoulder presses as well as all back exercises involve the elbow. So the elbow has little time to recover between two workouts.

Once you have elbow pain, it is very difficult to get rid of it.

This problem is not the result of chance or bad luck. It is the cumulative effect of three types of training mistakes:

Triceps brachii; medial head attaches under the tendinous part of the triceps brachii distal tendon — Humerus — Head of the radius — Radius — Ulna

Damaged triceps tendon — Triceps brachii tendon — Olecranon — Osteophyte causing weakness

⚠ Genetic predisposition, associated with intense and repetitive triceps work, can cause inflammation with an osteophyte (bone spur) at the base of the triceps brachii tendon. This problem weakens the tendon, and it could later tear during heavy work.

Neglecting the Valgus

Not taking your valgus into account is the first mistake. If your valgus affects the trajectory of biceps curls, it will also affect the contraction of the antagonist muscle. Using a straight bar for triceps work can place the elbow in a delicate position because your hand movement is restricted. It is better to use EZ bars or dumbbells or to do unilateral work with a cable pulley.

Should You Straighten Your Arms During Triceps Work?

The ability to extend the arms varies from person to person. Some people cannot completely straighten their arms; at best, their arms stay slightly bent. During triceps exercises, the less you can straighten your arms, the more you need to keep them under continuous tension and avoid exaggerating the contraction. Otherwise, you can develop elbow problems.

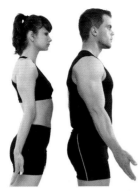

But for others, overextending the arm can allow it to go behind the body. This is called elbow recurvatum. In this case, instead of being aligned with the humerus, the ulna forms an angle. This anatomical peculiarity is more common in women than in men.

If you have elbow recurvatum you will easily be able to develop your triceps because you have a wider range of motion. So it is possible to shorten your triceps more during contraction as long as you do not feel any pain in the elbow.

Using Bars That Are Too Thin

In weightlifting, the diameter of the bars is about 1 inch (2.5 cm). Since this diameter is standard, it costs less for the manufacturers to produce. But this size is far from optimal for working the triceps. With a thin bar, the triceps is not as strong and the elbow is subject to greater mechanical stress.

A thicker bar (about 2 inches, or 5 cm) is better for transmitting hand strength to the triceps and thereby increasing their power. In addition, elbows endure less stress.

To take advantage of this double benefit, hold a sponge in your hand (its thickness will depend on the size of your hands) to increase the diameter of the bar.

HYGROMA OR BURSITIS

The sign of a hygroma is a swollen elbow. It is painful to the touch and when working out. The bump you see is, in fact, an accumulation of serous fluid in the bursa. The bursa is normally relatively flat. Its purpose is to facilitate the sliding of the triceps tendon on the bone. The swelling is the result of repeated microtraumas and lack of recovery time. The bursa becomes irritated and produces too much fluid, making the elbow swell. To reduce inflammation, apply ice and do not do any exercises involving the elbow. Since this type of pain is persistent and frequently recurring, we recommend that you pay close attention to this problem. Even if it seems fully healed, it is wise to minimize elbow trauma by eliminating any exercises that require bars, dumbbells, or machines and switch to cable exercises using a small range of motion. Decreasing the range of motion will reduce stress on the elbow by decreasing both the stretching and contraction phases (so you will not straighten your arm completely).

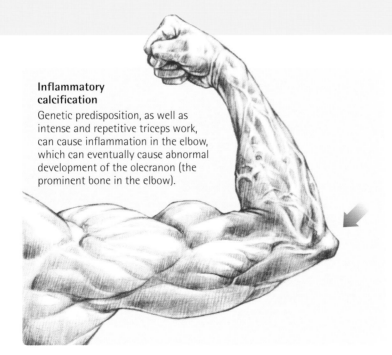

Inflammatory calcification
Genetic predisposition, as well as intense and repetitive triceps work, can cause inflammation in the elbow, which can eventually cause abnormal development of the olecranon (the prominent bone in the elbow).

⚠️ A hygroma can become infected and cause complications that compromise your ability to exercise. So it is important not to force things.

2 Types of Triceps Tears

There are three types of triceps tears:

Tears in the Tendon of the Long Head

The long head of the triceps is recruited in all exercises for the back and for the back of the shoulder. By cheating too much or by straightening your arms during pull-ups, you risk a partial tear in the tendon that attaches the long head to the shoulder blade.

To prevent this frequent but easily avoidable injury, we recommend that you
- warm up the triceps before working the back and the back of the shoulder,
- do not completely straighten your arms during any kind of pull-up exercise so that the exercise will not affect the triceps too much, and
- do specific stretches at the beginning of your workouts (see page 103).

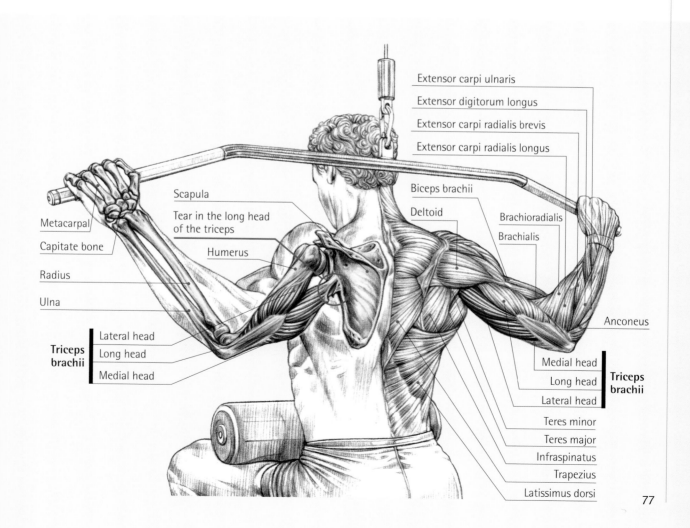

Extensor carpi ulnaris
Extensor digitorum longus
Extensor carpi radialis brevis
Extensor carpi radialis longus

Scapula
Tear in the long head of the triceps

Biceps brachii
Deltoid
Brachioradialis
Brachialis

Metacarpal
Capitate bone
Humerus

Radius

Ulna

Anconeus

Triceps brachii
Lateral head
Long head
Medial head

Medial head
Long head
Lateral head
Triceps brachii

Teres minor
Teres major
Infraspinatus
Trapezius
Latissimus dorsi

77

Tear in the Tendon Attachment

Unlike a tear in the lower biceps, which recovers more or less after an operation, a tear in the lower tendon attachment of the triceps will always leave a visible depression in the muscle.

This kind of tear occurs because of
- an extreme stretch of the triceps,
- frequent use of heavy weights,
- overusing weights and dumbbells and neglecting to alternate those workouts with less traumatic cable pulley workouts.

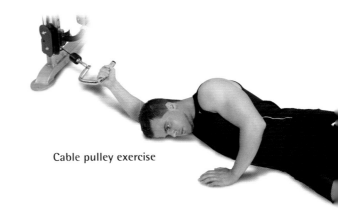

Cable pulley exercise

Tear in the distal tendon of the triceps

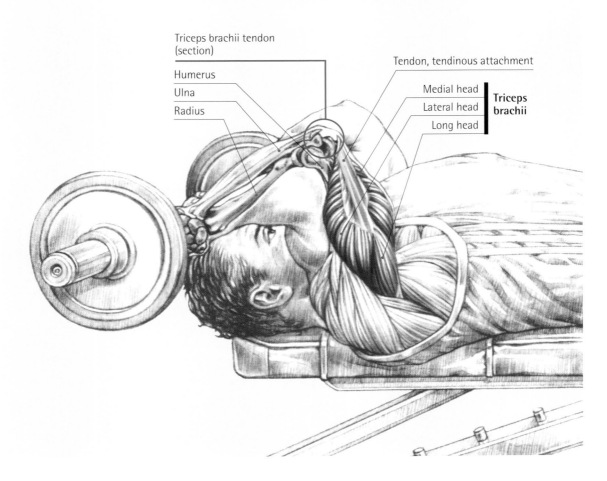

Triceps brachii tendon (section)

Humerus

Ulna

Radius

Tendon, tendinous attachment

Medial head

Lateral head — **Triceps brachii**

Long head

Progressive Degeneration of the Medial Head

In the lower part of the triceps, the small muscle fibers of the medial head insert directly on the humerus and under the tendinous attachment of the triceps. These fibers are very vulnerable and can be destroyed because of repeated inflammation of the triceps tendon. This degeneration ends up creating a depression on the inside of the arm between the muscle and the elbow, which makes it look like the muscles are getting shorter.

This pathology is more aesthetically displeasing than physically painful. Unfortunately, the damage cannot be reversed.

A depression just above the elbow, at the back of the arm, is also noted in more serious pathologies such as a rupture of the triceps tendon, because these fibers are the first ones affected by a triceps tear near the elbow.

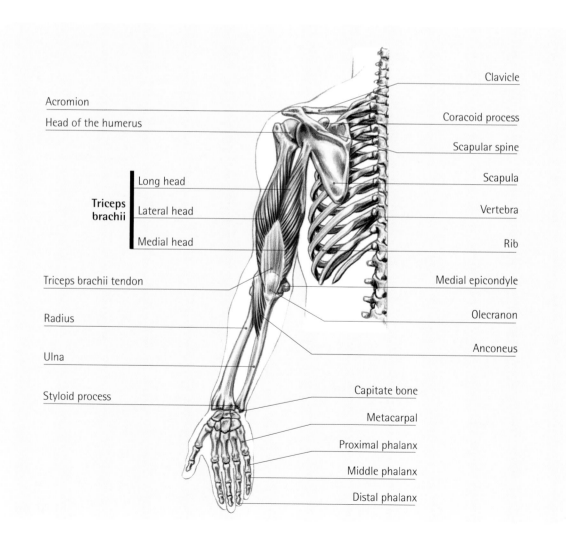

Acromion

Head of the humerus

Triceps brachii — Long head

Triceps brachii — Lateral head

Triceps brachii — Medial head

Triceps brachii tendon

Radius

Ulna

Styloid process

Clavicle

Coracoid process

Scapular spine

Scapula

Vertebra

Rib

Medial epicondyle

Olecranon

Anconeus

Capitate bone

Metacarpal

Proximal phalanx

Middle phalanx

Distal phalanx

UNDERSTANDING FOREARM AND WRIST PATHOLOGIES

As if developing your arms was not difficult enough already, many people who do strength training suffer from wrist and forearm problems. These injuries do not happen by chance; they have well-defined causes.

Factors That Predispose You to Forearm Pain

There are two groups of risk factors that predispose people to forearm or wrist pain:

1. Certain body types have joints, tendons, and muscles that are more vulnerable:
-   Pronounced elbow valgus
-   Hyperpronation
-   Small brachioradialis muscle
-   Long forearms with short muscles
-   Thin wrists that offer a small contact surface with the hand, increasing the tension per square inch
2. Classic training errors exacerbate these risks:
-   Not warming up the forearms before strength training or athletic workouts.
-   Not strengthening the extensor muscles in the wrist, brachioradialis, or supinator muscles.
-   Performing curls with weights that are too heavy.
-   Using straight bars during curls, triceps extensions, and back exercises. This causes too great of a stretch in the muscles responsible for wrist rotation (supinator muscles). The heavier the bars are, the more this overstretching can lead to microtraumas and inflammation.
-   An excessive range of motion in wrist movements during hand extension and flexion exercises, especially during the stretching phase.
-   Using bars that are too thin and that do not stabilize the wrist sufficiently.

Tendinitis in Muscles Attaching to the Epicondyles

The most common problem affecting the forearm is epicondylitis.

At the elbow, the lateral extremities of the humerus form two bumps called epicondyles (*epi* means on the condyle, that is, the joint). The medial epicondyle is the most prominent and is located on the pinky side of the arm when the hand is supinated. Some of the wrist flexor muscles attach to it.

The lateral epicondyle is smaller and is located on the thumb side of the arm when the hand is supinated. Some of the wrist extensor muscles attach to it.

Since they are used often in daily life and in sports, the muscle attachment sites at the epicondyles are frequently affected by inflammation and tendinitis. These can be both painful and debilitating.

Pain in the muscles attached to the lateral epicondyle is commonly called tennis elbow. When the muscles attaching to the medial epicondyle are affected, it is called golfer's elbow. It affects not only golfers but also athletes who do shot put.

In sports requiring arm movements, about 50 percent of pain is from tennis elbow. Tennis elbow is twice as common as golfer's elbow and is also more debilitating.

Unlike classic tendinitis affecting the central part of a tendon, epicondylitis occurs more often at the tendon–bone junction. Repeatedly overstretching creates microtraumas where the muscles attach to the bone, and this damage requires a great deal of time to heal.

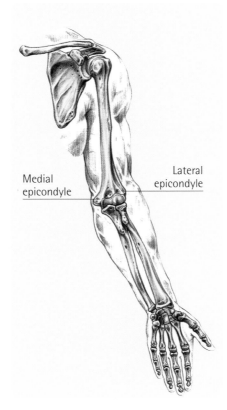

Medial epicondyle

Lateral epicondyle

One of the most common causes of medial epicondylitis is curls or pull-ups with heavy weights. The more you lift the weight, the more you pull on the wrist and finger flexor muscles. This extra tension can damage the tendons.

Following are the causes of lateral epicondylitis:

1. Poorly controlled repetitive pronosupination movements during dumbbell curls. It can become very painful to rotate the wrist during these curls. Hammer curls also become impossible. In this specific case, to keep from losing volume in the biceps muscle, the solution is to do light curls with a straight bar, which avoids pronosupination.
2. Stretching the wrist extensor muscles during curls. The more you lift the bar, the more you stretch the wrist extensors. This is even truer if you are a hyperpronator using a straight bar for curls.
3. Doing snatches in a row. In the negative phase, when the exercise is performed abruptly, the extensor muscles suffer abuse.

Prevent Pain in the Forearms and Wrists

You can avoid these injuries by following 11 simple rules:

1. Warm up the forearms well before a workout, whether the workout is strength training or playing a sport. Do at least 1 long set (50 repetitions) of extensions plus 1 long set of wrist curls.
2. Strengthen the forearms using specific exercises (see "Exercises for the Forearms" on page 104 and "Advanced Exercises for the Forearms" on page 141).
3. Correct any strength imbalances between the flexors and the extensors in the forearms.
4. Do specific work for the pronosupinator and supinator muscles in the hand (see "Advanced Exercises for the Forearms" on page 141).
5. Avoid extreme stretching of the wrist, especially during forearm exercises in a lengthened position.
6. Do not straighten the arm with your hands in a supinated position during biceps, chest, or back exercises.

7. Allow your forearms more time to recover because these muscles are used in almost every strength training exercise, in many athletic activities, and in daily life.
8. Protect your wrists by wearing wrist guards when using heavy weights for curls, bench press, and push-ups.
9. Avoid rotating your hands during dumbbell curls (see "Exercises for the Biceps" on page 88).
10. Use a thick sponge to increase the diameter of the bars for biceps as well as for triceps exercises. Having your hand open wider reduces the stretch on the extensors and minimizes trauma to the forearm.
11. Avoid bar snatches unless you can keep your wrists very rigid.

Goals of a Strength Training Program for Preventing Wrist Injuries

The goals of preventive strength training include the following:

- Strengthen the flexors and extensors.
- Correct strength imbalances between two antagonist muscle groups.
- Increase their co-contraction coordination.
- Increase the speed of muscle contraction in the forearms.

The goal is to be able to hold the wrist as rigid as possible during heavy work. This rigidity happens because of synchronized co-contraction of the flexors and extensors. The rigidity helps avoid micromovements that are the source of problems in powerlifting or combat sports. For example, when you throw a punch, if your wrist vacillates upon impact, the punch will not be effective and you will hurt yourself. If your fist stays rigid, the punch will be more effective, and the shock to your wrist is distributed over a greater surface area.

In boxing, a good punch is thrown in 50 to 250 milliseconds. But a nontrained muscle needs 600 to 800 milliseconds to reach its maximum strength. So it is essential that the speed of muscle contraction be as fast as possible. It would be pointless for the rigidity to appear after the impact because the muscles were too slow. This speed is provided through a combination of heavy work and lighter, more explosive training.

Another example is the heavy bench press. If the wrist is not rigid enough, the transmission of strength from the arms to the bar decreases and the chance of twisting the wrist increases.

PART 3

The Exercises

1

Beginning Exercises

WORK YOUR ARMS AT HOME WITH LITTLE EQUIPMENT

Here are the simplest arm exercises that you can do at home with little equipment. You can also do them at the gym.

However, just because they are simple exercises does not mean they are not effective. You do not need ultrasophisticated machines to build your arms. More than equipment, your desire and perseverance will get you powerful and well-developed arms.

It is always possible to train without equipment, but basic materials will increase the number of exercises you can do and make those exercises more effective. Ideally, you should get a pair of dumbbells, a pull-up bar, and some elastic bands.

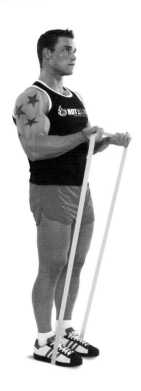

Dumbbells

Adjustable dumbbells are available in any sporting goods store. A 25-pound set costs about $20. Ideally, you should have two. Then, as you progress, you can buy additional weights as needed. The good thing about dumbbells is that you can increase the difficulty of the exercises you do so you continue to make progress. If you always train with the same weight (your body weight, for example), even if you increase the number of repetitions and sets, you will quickly reach a plateau. In strength training, everything is based on the principle of overload. Dumbbells are the best way to obtain this overload.

Pull-Up Bar

This is a removable bar that you can attach to a door frame or between two walls in a hallway. After you use it, you can easily store it out of sight. There are short bars (less than 3 feet, or 1 m) and longer bars (up to 4 feet, or 1.2 m). If you have the room, choose the longer bar, because it will allow you do a wider variety of exercises.

Elastic Bands

Elastic bands or cords are available in any sporting goods store. The advantage of bands is that they provide rather high resistance without actually weighing anything. Bands are easy to transport and store at home. Ideally, you should have several sizes so that you can easily vary your resistance.

The resistance provided by bands is very different from the resistance provided by a dumbbell. The more you pull on a band, the more the resistance increases. However, if you lift a 25-pound dumbbell, it will always weigh 25 pounds whether you are at the beginning, middle, or end of the exercise.

1 Pull-Up

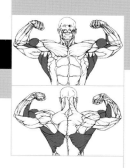

This exercise works the biceps, the forearm flexors, and the back muscles. It is the only true classic compound exercise for the biceps. Unilateral work is next to impossible except for very small or exceptionally strong people.

Grab the bar with supinated hands (pinky fingers facing each other). Your hands should be about shoulder-width apart. If it does not hurt your wrists, you can even move your hands closer together. The closer the grip, the harder the biceps have to work.

Pull yourself up using the strength of your biceps ❶. You do not need to go all the way to the bar. You will reach the height of the movement when the biceps are well contracted. Hold the position for 1 second before slowly lowering yourself down.

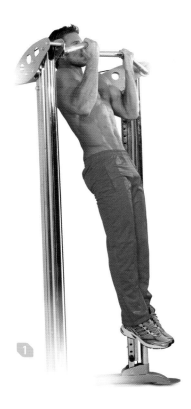

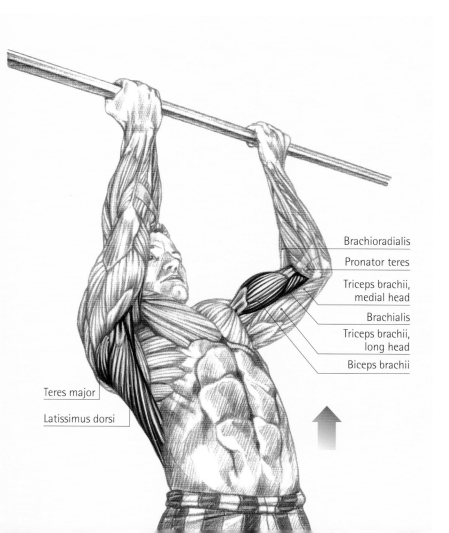

Brachioradialis
Pronator teres
Triceps brachii, medial head
Brachialis
Triceps brachii, long head
Biceps brachii
Teres major
Latissimus dorsi

HELPFUL HINTS

Unlike back exercises in which you try to work the biceps as little as possible, here the objective is to recruit them as much as possible. You are not trying to contract the muscles in the back. To do this, lean slightly backward and bring the bar as close to the bottom of your neck as you can.

85

ADVANTAGES

Pull-ups are the only classic compound exercise for the biceps. They stretch the biceps near the shoulder while contracting it near the elbow. Pull-ups exploit the length–tension relationship perfectly, which makes them an excellent exercise for quickly building up your arms.

DISADVANTAGES

Unfortunately, not everyone can do a pull-up. To compensate for lack of strength, you have four choices:

1. Rest your feet on the floor or a chair to lighten your weight.
2. Do only the lowering part of the exercise (just the negative phase) and use a chair to go back up.
3. Position the bar 3 feet (1 m) high and do pull-ups with your body parallel to the floor with your feet touching the floor.
4. At first, only do half pull-ups (the end of the exercise) and go a little lower each time you work out.

NOTE

Pull-ups allow you to work the back and the arms simultaneously, which will save time during your workout.

RISKS

⚠ As in all pulling exercises, you should never straighten your arms completely when your hands are supinated (pinky fingers next to each other) because this puts the biceps, especially the short head, in a position where it could tear. This is especially true if you are using a straight pull-up bar.

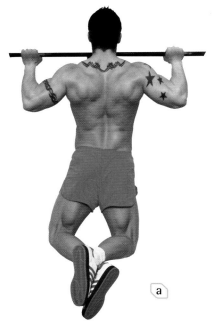

a

Variations

(a) To work the brachioradialis muscle more, use a pronated grip (thumbs facing each other). The biceps works less, so you will not be as strong in this position.

(b) To target the brachialis, use a neutral grip (thumbs toward your torso). To do this, you will need a bar that allows you to use a narrow parallel grip. This is the easiest position for pull-ups since your arms are strongest when using a neutral grip.

(c) Once pull-ups become too easy, you can add weight.

⚠ Out of convenience, this exercise is often done using a straight pull-up bar. However, with your arms in the air, your ability to rotate your wrist is severely limited when the hand is supinated. Most people will have to force their joints to grasp the bar. This restriction can cause problems in the wrist, forearm, biceps, or shoulder. It is better to use an EZ bar, which is more natural for the wrist, especially if you hyperpronate (see next page).

DEGREES OF ELBOW EXTENSION

The ability to straighten the arms varies from person to person. Some people cannot completely straighten their arms. If this is the case for you, you should not force the stretch and allow gravity to pull your arms straight during pull-ups or curls.

The smaller the degree of extension in your arms, the more you should avoid straightening them during biceps exercises.

People with elbow recurvatum have a greater range of motion in exercises. But we do not recommend using it because, even with recurvatum, the more the arms are straightened, the greater the chance of tearing the biceps when the hand is supinated in curls or pull-ups.

When the arms are lifted, the pectoralis major presses on the biceps, primarily the short head. This tension is even stronger when the hands are supinated. It is not surprising that tears in the short head of the biceps frequently happen during pull-ups using a supinated grip.

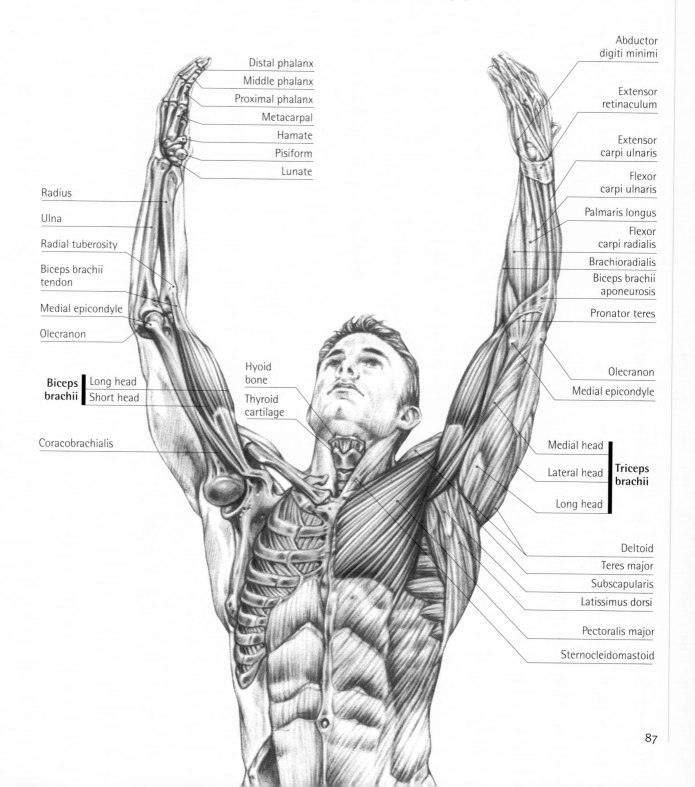

Distal phalanx
Middle phalanx
Proximal phalanx
Metacarpal
Hamate
Pisiform
Lunate

Radius
Ulna
Radial tuberosity
Biceps brachii tendon
Medial epicondyle
Olecranon

Biceps brachii | Long head
Short head

Coracobrachialis

Hyoid bone
Thyroid cartilage

Abductor digiti minimi
Extensor retinaculum
Extensor carpi ulnaris
Flexor carpi ulnaris
Palmaris longus
Flexor carpi radialis
Brachioradialis
Biceps brachii aponeurosis
Pronator teres

Olecranon
Medial epicondyle

Medial head
Lateral head
Long head
Triceps brachii

Deltoid
Teres major
Subscapularis
Latissimus dorsi
Pectoralis major
Sternocleidomastoid

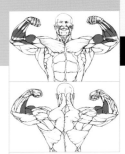

BEGINNING EXERCISES FOR THE BICEPS
2 Supinated Curl

This is an isolation exercise for the biceps. It also works the brachialis and brachioradialis muscles to varying degrees. It is better to work unilaterally if large biceps are your main goal.

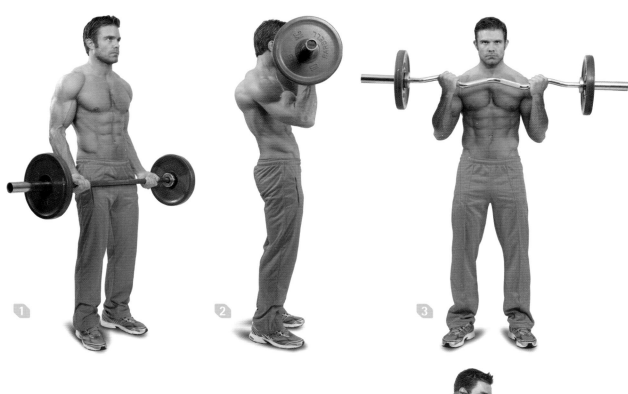

🔹 **With a bar:** Grab the bar (straight or twisted) using a supinated grip (pinky fingers facing each other) **1**. Use your biceps to bend your arms. Raise the bar as high as you can **2**. Hold the contracted position for 1 second while squeezing your forearms against your biceps as much as possible **3**. Slowly lower the bar without straightening your arms too much in the lengthened position.

🔹 **With dumbbells 4:** Grab the dumbbells and keep your hands in a neutral position. Rotate the wrists to bring the thumbs toward the outside, and bend your arms using your biceps. Bring the dumbbells as high as possible. You can lift your elbows slightly, but do not overdo it. Hold the contracted position for 1 second and then slowly lower to the starting position.

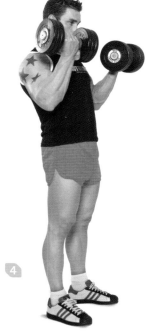

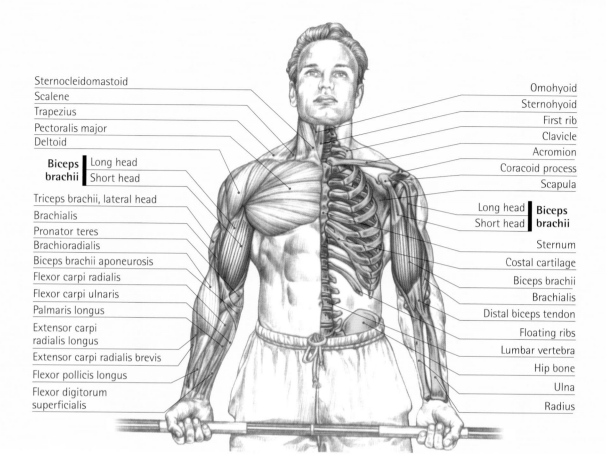

Sternocleidomastoid
Scalene
Trapezius
Pectoralis major
Deltoid
Biceps brachii | Long head
Short head
Triceps brachii, lateral head
Brachialis
Pronator teres
Brachioradialis
Biceps brachii aponeurosis
Flexor carpi radialis
Flexor carpi ulnaris
Palmaris longus
Extensor carpi radialis longus
Extensor carpi radialis brevis
Flexor pollicis longus
Flexor digitorum superficialis

Omohyoid
Sternohyoid
First rib
Clavicle
Acromion
Coracoid process
Scapula
Long head | **Biceps brachii**
Short head
Sternum
Costal cartilage
Biceps brachii
Brachialis
Distal biceps tendon
Floating ribs
Lumbar vertebra
Hip bone
Ulna
Radius

ADVANTAGES

This is a good way to isolate the biceps. Dumbbells allow the wrists to move freely, which prevents the kinds of injuries that can happen when using a straight bar or a machine.

DISADVANTAGES

This exercise does not exploit the length-tension relationship. The temptation to cheat in this exercise is stronger than for other exercises. This can work against you by preventing the biceps from contracting well. Do more forced repetitions because they are not as dangerous.

RISKS

⚠ If you cheat too much by swinging your torso from front to back so that you can use heavier weights or do a few more repetitions, you could injure your back. To learn to do this exercise with strict form, begin by standing with your back against a wall. Given the risks, do not use a straight bar too often.

⚠ When using dumbbells, you can either rotate the wrists on every repetition or keep your hands supinated. Use the position that feels most natural for your arms. If you choose to use a pronated grip, then you should never straighten your arm all the way (especially with heavy weights) because you could tear your biceps. This will not be a problem if you use a neutral grip in the lengthened position. However, we do not recommend rotation (see page 91).

Variations

(a) Use a band in addition to regular weights. At failure, release the band so you can do a few more repetitions.

(b) A wider grip on the bar will work the short head more. A narrow grip will recruit the long head a little more.

(c) Drag curls using a bar: The principle is to pull the elbow gradually back as you raise the bar so that it is constantly touching the torso. The advantage of this variation is that it lightly stretches the upper part of the biceps as the lower part contracts, which almost makes it into a compound exercise. Athletes who have trouble doing curls because of long forearms will enjoy drag curls because they eliminate that obstacle by pulling the elbow backward.

(d) When using dumbbells, you can work either one arm at a time or both arms. You will be strongest when you work only one arm at a time.

(e) You can do dumbbell curls while sitting or standing. One possible strategy is to begin the exercise sitting down so you can use strict form. At failure, stand up so that you can do a few more repetitions by cheating a bit.

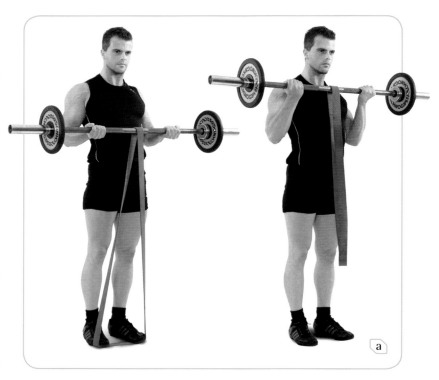

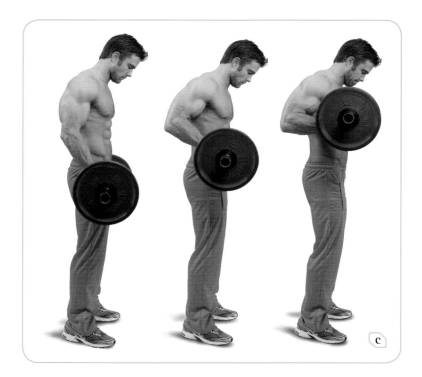

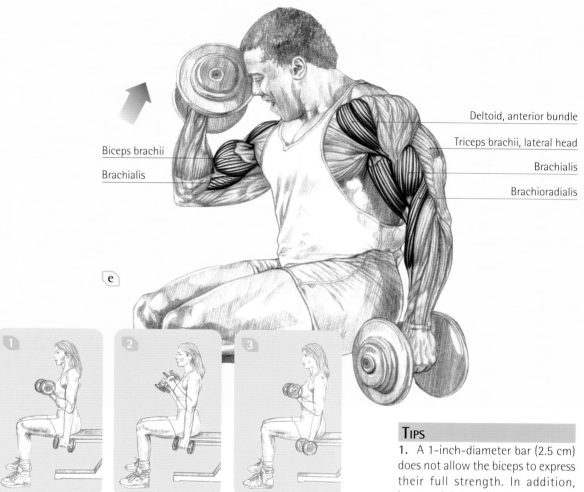

Biceps brachii

Brachialis

Deltoid, anterior bundle

Triceps brachii, lateral head

Brachialis

Brachioradialis

Three ways to do dumbbell curls:
1. Mainly works the biceps and the brachialis
2. Works the brachioradialis intensely
3. Mainly works the biceps

SHOULD YOU ROTATE THE WRIST WHEN USING DUMBBELLS?

Here are four advantages of rotating the wrist during dumbbell curls:
- It makes it easier to lower the dumbbell so that you do not hit your thigh.
- It creates a more physiological movement for the arm.
- It works the biceps and the brachialis simultaneously.
- It reduces the risk of tears in the biceps when the arm is straight.
  But the disadvantages of rotation outweigh the benefits:
- The isolation of the biceps work is not as good because the brachialis performs almost half of the exercise.
- The isolation of the brachialis work is not optimal because the biceps prevents its recruitment during the entire upper part of the exercise.
- Rotation can damage the humeroradial joint.
- Rotation causes problems such as tennis elbow.

TIPS

1. A 1-inch-diameter bar (2.5 cm) does not allow the biceps to express their full strength. In addition, because it is too thin, it encourages problems in the forearms. A thicker bar (about 2 inches) will transmit the hands' strength to the biceps better, which augments the biceps' power. Use a sponge (the thickness will depend on the size of your hands) to increase the diameter of the bar.

2. Between sets, shake each biceps using the opposite hand to relax it and accelerate recovery.

3. With adjustable dumbbells, place the weights a little off center on the bar. Put the weights as close to the side of your pinky finger as possible. This way, you will not hit your thigh or torso with the bar.

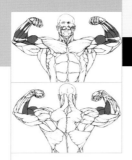

BEGINNING EXERCISES FOR THE BICEPS
3 Hammer Curl

This isolation exercise targets the brachialis and brachioradialis muscles but does not work the biceps as much as curls using a pronated grip. You can do it unilaterally.

NOTES

The need to do this exercise will be dictated by the size of your brachialis muscle. If it is the same size as your biceps, then this exercise will not be useful. If your brachialis muscle is underdeveloped compared to your biceps, then doing hammer curls makes a lot of sense. Hammer curls can even replace classic curls until your brachialis muscle has caught up to your biceps.

Grab a dumbbell with your hand in the neutral position (thumb pointing up, as if you were grabbing a hammer; hence the name of this exercise).

Bend your arm and keep your thumb pointing up. Lift the dumbbell as high as possible. To do this, you can pull your elbow back in slightly, but be careful not to move it too much. Hold the contracted position for 1 second.

Slowly lower back to the starting position. Since you are using a neutral grip, you can straighten your arm almost completely without any problems.

HELPFUL HINTS

In the neutral position, your arm is stronger than when your hand is supinated. So it is normal to be able to use heavier weights with hammer curls than with classic curls. You just have to be careful not to reduce your range of motion because you picked a weight that is too heavy.

Variations

a You can do this exercise while sitting or standing. One possible strategy is to begin the exercise while seated. At failure, stand up so that you can do a few more repetitions by cheating a bit.

b You can either lift both dumbbells at the same time or lift one after the other. You will be strongest in the latter version.

c If you do seated concentration curls or use a Scott curl bench, you will double the work of the brachialis.

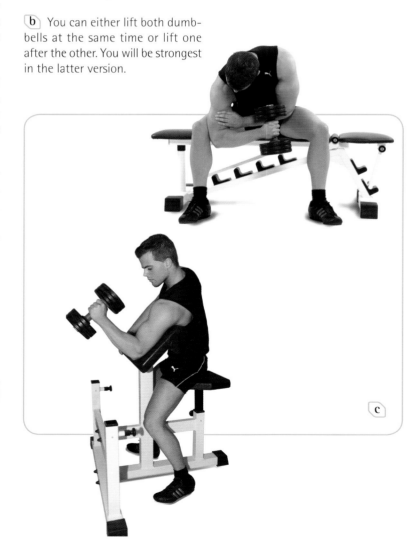

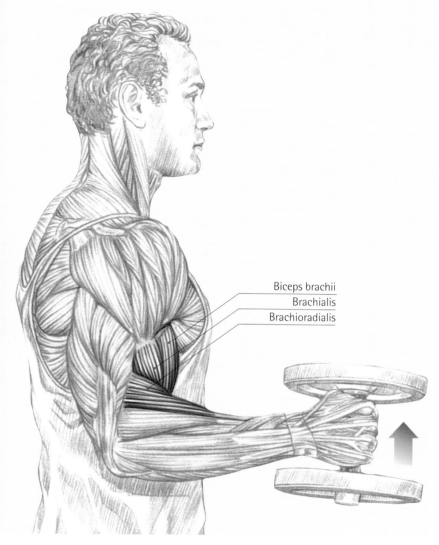

Biceps brachii
Brachialis
Brachioradialis

If you are a beginner, you can do either regular curls or hammer curls. However, you should not do both during the same workout. You can alternate a workout with hammer curls and a workout with regular curls. The relationship between the two will be determined by the development of your biceps and brachialis muscles, respectively. Another alternative is to do classic curls until you reach failure and then finish in a superset with hammer curls.

ADVANTAGES

The strengthening of the forearm provided by hammer curls helps prevent pain that frequently develops during strength training. As with all curls done unilaterally, at the end of a set you can use your free hand to do a few forced repetitions.

DISADVANTAGES

Hammer curls are not necessarily useful in a strength training program because classic curls and pull-ups are already working the brachialis muscle.

RISKS

⚠ Be careful of your back and your wrists, especially when using heavy weights.

d Using a weight plate with a handhold will change the lever compared to using a dumbbell, and this will improve the exercise.

93

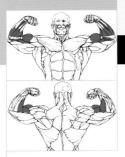

BEGINNING EXERCISES FOR THE BICEPS
4 Concentration Curl

This isolation exercise works the brachialis muscle a bit better and the biceps a bit less than classic curls. It especially isolates the interior of the biceps. It is done only unilaterally.

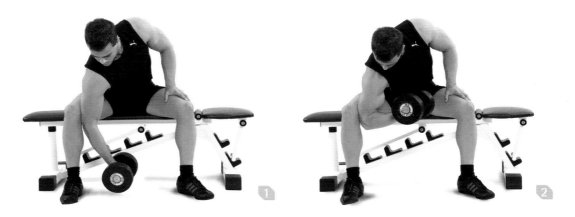

🔹 While seated, grab a dumbbell with one supinated hand (thumb away from your body).

🔹 Place your triceps against the inside of your thigh **1**. Bend the arm using your biceps. Lift the dumbbell as high as possible without lifting your elbow **2**. Hold the contracted position for 1 second while squeezing your forearm against your biceps as much as possible.

🔹 Slowly lower back to the starting position. You must still avoid straightening your arm completely.

HELPFUL HINTS

This exercise is supposed to work the peak of the biceps, giving it a rounder form. This is because of the additional recruitment of the brachialis. By pushing the biceps up, the brachialis tends to alter the form of the biceps slightly.

Variation

You can use a supinated grip or a hammer grip (thumb pointing up). The latter version will force the brachialis to work even harder.

NOTE

Begin your set with concentration curls (supinated or neutral grip); at failure, change to normal curls so you can get a few additional repetitions.

ADVANTAGES

By working the brachialis muscle a bit more than classic curls do, concentration curls help to balance the development of the brachialis muscle compared to the biceps.

DISADVANTAGES

This exercise is not the best for increasing muscle mass. It is popular mostly because it is relatively easy to do. Since it is done unilaterally, it takes more time.

RISKS

⚠ To press your triceps against your thigh, you have to round your back. To protect your back, press your free hand on your thigh to relieve pressure from your spinal column.

94

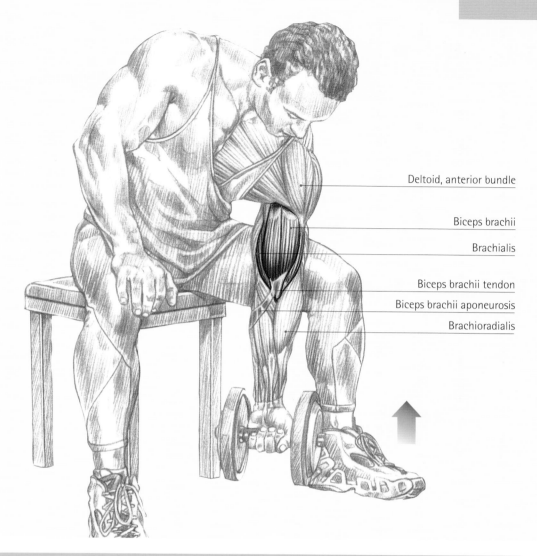

Deltoid, anterior bundle

Biceps brachii

Brachialis

Biceps brachii tendon

Biceps brachii aponeurosis

Brachioradialis

5 Biceps Stretch

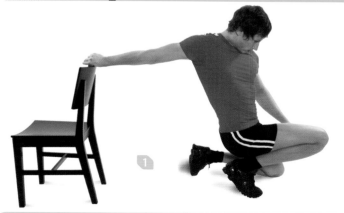

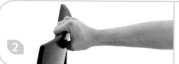

To stretch the biceps, put one hand on the back of a chair. Turn your back very slowly toward the chair 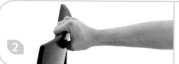.

Rotate your wrist from top to bottom to stretch both heads of the biceps 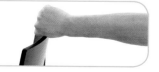. Do not make jerky movements, because your muscle is in a very vulnerable position.

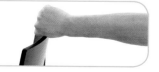
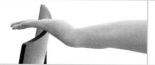

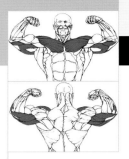

1 Narrow Push-Up

This is a compound exercise for the triceps, shoulders, and chest.
Unilateral work is possible, but only for extremely light people.

ADVANTAGES

It is easy to adjust the resistance. If your body weight is too great, begin doing push-ups on your knees rather than on your feet so that you can gain strength. In the same way, at the end of a set, if you do not have enough energy to do any more regular push-ups, continue doing the exercise on your knees so you can do a few more repetitions.

Other than narrow-grip bench press and dips, push-ups are the only triceps exercise that exploits the length–tension relationship in the long head.

DISADVANTAGES

It is not easy to focus on the triceps during push-ups. In addition, push-ups do not necessarily work well for every person's anatomy. If you have long arms, you will have great difficulty without any guarantee of results.

Push-ups are not the end goal. Strength training should not be a select club for people who can do push-ups or a circus for people to show off crazy push-up variations.

The dumbbell exercises that we describe next are a more reliable way to target the triceps.

Stretch out facing the floor with your hands on the floor. Your hands should be shoulder-width apart at most. If you do not feel any pain in your wrists, you can use an even narrower grip. You can place your feet however far apart as is comfortable for you.

Straighten your arms to raise your body using the strength of your triceps as much as possible. Once your arms are straight, lower your body slowly.

HELPFUL HINTS

To better target the outside of the triceps, turn your hands slightly inward.

RISKS

⚠ Arching your back will make this exercise easier, but it could compromise your spine.

All wrists are not made to be bent at a 90-degree angle. So that you do not damage your forearms, you can use special push-up bars, which are available in sporting goods stores. They increase the range of motion of the exercise while preventing the wrist from twisting too much.

Variations

a Hands close together: The closer together you place your hands, the more the triceps work, taking away some of the work from the chest.

b Hands far apart: The farther apart you place your hands, the more the chest will work. You will also be stronger, but the triceps will not work as much. One possible combination is to start the exercise with your hands close together. At failure, move your hands farther apart to compensate for your fatigued triceps by letting your chest do more of the work.

c To add resistance, put a band around your back and hold it in your hands. At first, wrap it only once around your back.

When you get stronger, you can wrap it twice around your back.

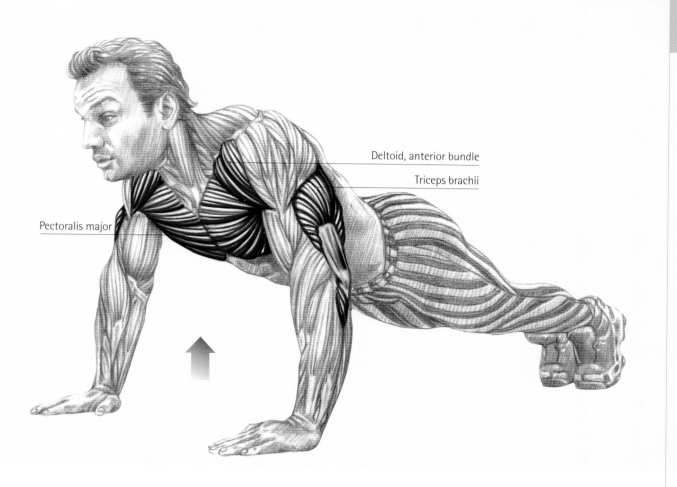

Pectoralis major

Deltoid, anterior bundle

Triceps brachii

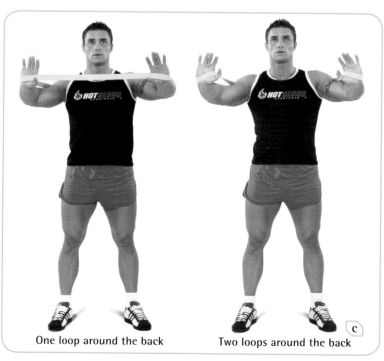

One loop around the back

Two loops around the back

c

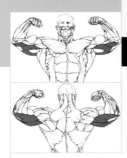

BEGINNING EXERCISES FOR THE TRICEPS
2 Seated or Standing Triceps Extension With Dumbbells

This is an isolation exercise for the triceps.
You can do it unilaterally.

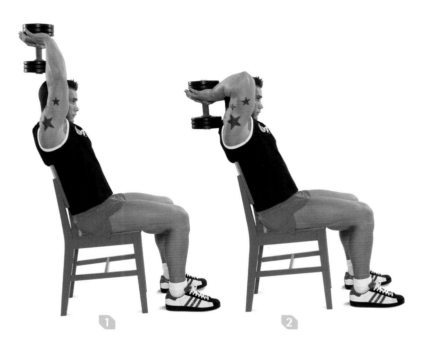

NOTES

Ideally, you should keep the elbow as high as possible and the arms close to your head. This is not always possible, because the ability to lift the arms varies from person to person. Some people cannot completely straighten their arms up in the air, and despite all their efforts their arms stay far from the head. If this is the case for you, then do not force things. Place the elbow where it is comfortable, even if it is far from your head.

ADVANTAGES

This exercise provides a good stretch in the long head. If you work unilaterally, then during the contraction, rotate your wrist toward the outside. Moving your pinky from the front toward the side will better target the outside head of the triceps.

DISADVANTAGES

The elbows are really worked during this exercise, so you must perform the exercise with control to avoid hurting them. If you have elbow pain, reduce the range of motion. This exercise does not really exploit the length–tension relationship in the triceps.

RISKS

⚠ When you work bilaterally, it is easy to let your back arch. Be careful not to bump your head with the dumbbell.

Sit or stand. Grab a dumbbell with both hands (for bilateral work) or with one hand (for unilateral work) **1**. Move the dumbbell behind your head, with your elbows and pinky fingers pointing toward the ceiling **2**.

Use your triceps to straighten your arms before bringing the weight back down.

HELPFUL HINTS

The range of motion is much greater when this exercise is done unilaterally rather than bilaterally, because the stretch is better and the contraction is more pronounced.

Variations

If you are working bilaterally, it is best to maintain continuous tension. This means that you never completely straighten your arms. However, if you are working unilaterally, you can straighten your arm so that you can really contract the triceps.

If you are working unilaterally, you can choose any hand position from a pronated to a neutral to a supinated grip. Choose the position that is most comfortable for your elbow.

3 Lying Triceps Extension With Dumbbells

This exercise targets the triceps. You can do it unilaterally.

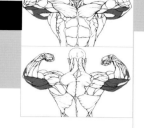

🔹 Lie on your back and grab the dumbbells. Lower them slowly behind your head with your hands in the neutral position (pinky fingers toward the ceiling). Stretch the triceps to its maximum without moving your arms too much. The elbows should remain pointing toward the ceiling.

🔹 Using your triceps, lift the weights ❶. Contract for 1 second before you lower the weights.

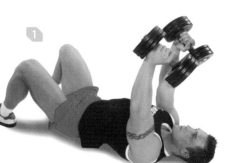

Variation

Even if you are working bilaterally, you can use one or two dumbbells. To learn the proper form, you should begin with just one dumbbell and hold it with both of your hands, as in the previous exercise. In this way, you will be able to control the weight better.

HELPFUL HINTS

You can bring the dumbbells behind your head or just to your ears. Choose where to stop based on what feels most natural for your elbows.

NOTE

Do not confuse this exercise with a pullover. At all times, the upper arms stay basically perpendicular to the floor.

ADVANTAGES

The back is protected when you are lying down.

Your form will also be better than when you do triceps extensions while in a seated or standing position.

Dumbbells allow you to vary the position of your hands by using a number of possible grips. Compared to using bars or machines, this freedom of movement in the wrist helps you feel the triceps more while protecting your elbows.

DISADVANTAGES

The elbows are worked hard during this exercise. You must perform the exercise with great control so that you do not injure them. The length-tension relationship of the muscle is not exploited as much as it should be for optimal effectiveness.

RISKS

⚠ Be careful not to bump your head with the dumbbells, especially if fatigue begins to affect your form.

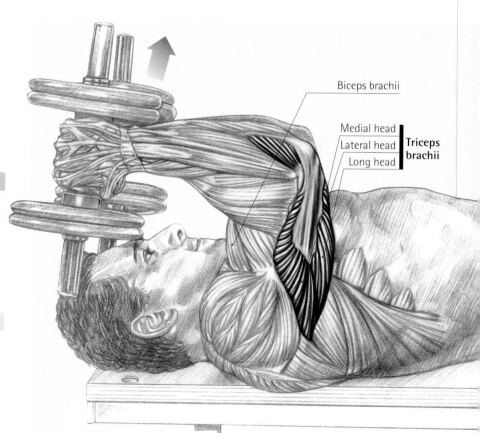

Biceps brachii

Medial head
Lateral head — Triceps brachii
Long head

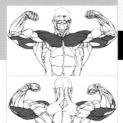

BEGINNING EXERCISES FOR THE TRICEPS
4 Reverse Dip

This is a compound exercise for the triceps, chest, and shoulders.
You cannot do it unilaterally.

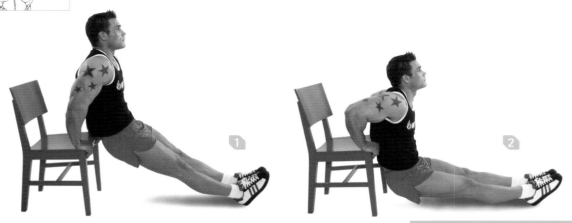

🖐 Turn your back to your bed or a chair and place your hands on the edge with pronated wrists (thumbs facing each other). Keep your legs straight out in front of you **1**.

🖐 Bend your arms to lower your body toward the floor, and then use your triceps to lift yourself back up **2**. You do not need to have a very large range of motion; about 20 inches (50 cm) should be enough.

HELPFUL HINTS
When you push on your triceps to lift yourself up, keep your head very straight and your eyes looking slightly toward the ceiling.

NOTES
When this exercise becomes too easy for you, put another chair or bench in front of you so that you can put your feet on it **3**. In this way, your triceps will have to move more of your body weight. One possible combination is to begin with your feet on a chair and then, at failure, finish the exercise with your feet on the floor so that you can get the maximum number of repetitions. If you want to increase the resistance further, put a weight on your thighs **4**.

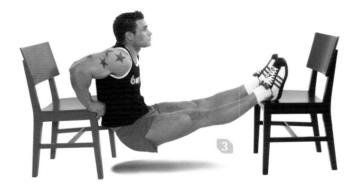

Variation

Vary the width of your hands as well as their orientation until you find the position that works best for your triceps muscles.

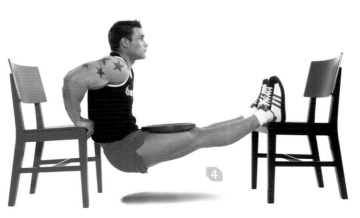

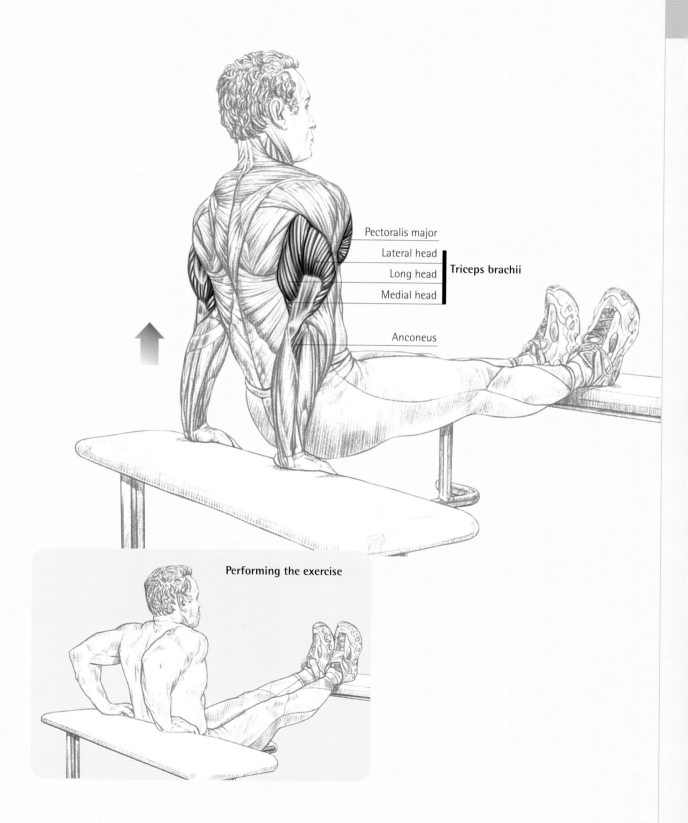

Pectoralis major

Lateral head
Long head   **Triceps brachii**
Medial head

Anconeus

Performing the exercise

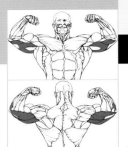

BEGINNING EXERCISES FOR THE TRICEPS

5 Triceps Kickback

This is an isolation exercise for the triceps.
It is best to do it unilaterally.

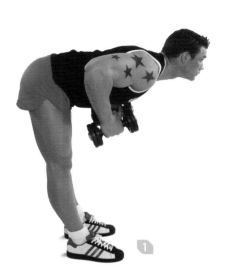

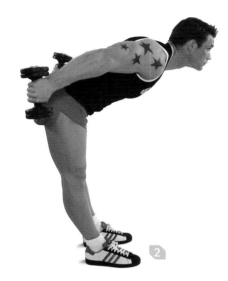

Lean forward and grab one or two dumbbells with your hands in the neutral position (thumbs pointing forward). Your upper arms should be glued to your sides and parallel to the floor while your forearms are bent to 90 degrees **1**.

HELPFUL HINTS
When your arms are extended, hold the contraction of the triceps as long as possible. In fact, unlike with other triceps exercises, you have to generate a lot of muscular tension to keep your arms extended during this exercise. Take full advantage of this characteristic.

NOTE
By turning your pinky finger slightly to the outside in the contracted position, you can better focus the work on the exterior of the triceps.

Using your triceps, straighten your arms **2**. Hold the contracted position for at least 1 second before lowering the weights.

Variations

a You can either keep the elbow toward the back or lift it a little toward the ceiling. For some people, this version helps in feeling the work of the triceps a little better.

b To accentuate the work of the triceps even more, lie on a decline bench (head on the lower part of the bench) so that your elbow points even more toward the ceiling.

c Using a cable pulley will increase the range of motion for this exercise.

ADVANTAGES
Of all triceps exercises, this one is the easiest on the elbow. You should be able to do these even if your elbow hurts when you do other triceps exercises. Note that if you do have pain, it is best to stop and let your elbow rest.

DISADVANTAGES
This exercise does not make use of the length–tension relationship of the muscle. Because there is little stretching in this exercise, you might have trouble feeling it.

RISKS
⚠ Working bilaterally involves the lower back, but when you work unilaterally, you can support your back by pressing your free hand on the thigh or the bench.

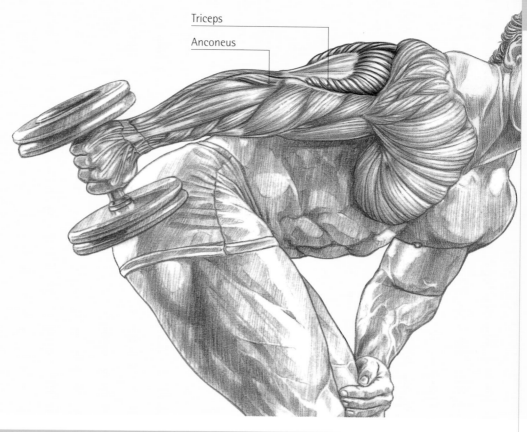

Triceps

Anconeus

6 Triceps Stretch

Stand up and lift your right arm so that your biceps is close to your head.

Use your left hand to bend your right arm as much as you can. Ideally, your right hand should touch your right shoulder.

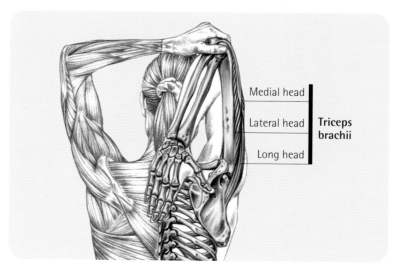

Medial head

Lateral head — **Triceps brachii**

Long head

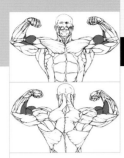

BEGINNING EXERCISES FOR THE FOREARMS

1 Reverse Curl

This isolation exercise targets the brachioradialis specifically, the brachialis to a lesser extent, and a little bit of the biceps.
Unilateral work is possible but not essential.

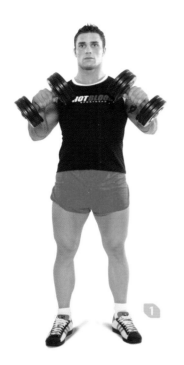

🖐 Grab an EZ bar or a pair of dumbbells using a pronated grip (thumbs facing each other).

🖐 Bend your arms to lift your hands as high as possible **1** **2**. Unlike other curls, do not lift your elbow during this exercise so that you can really maintain the contraction of the brachioradialis. Hold the contraction for 1 second before lowering the weight to the starting position.

HELPFUL HINTS

Unless you are a hyperpronator, the straight bar could be uncomfortable for your wrists.

Generally, an EZ bar will be more comfortable.

If you have both a pronounced valgus and are a hypersupinator, even EZ bars could be uncomfortable. In this case, dumbbells are the best choice. The arm is in a relatively weak position, so you must use considerably less weight for reverse curls than for other kinds of curls.

NOTE

With dumbbells, you can begin the exercise with reverse curls. At failure, turn the wrist a little and continue the exercise doing hammer curls.

ADVANTAGES

A strong brachioradialis will provide strength during curls and pull-ups while at the same time preventing triceps injuries.

DISADVANTAGES

In an ideal world, this exercise would be superfluous because working the biceps and the back intensely should help develop the brachioradialis muscle.

RISKS

⚠ Be careful of your wrists. Always keep your thumb a little higher than your pinky finger so you can prevent the forearm from twisting too much.

NOTE

The size of your brachioradialis will determine whether or not you need to do this exercise. If it is already well developed from doing other curls, then this exercise will not be especially useful.

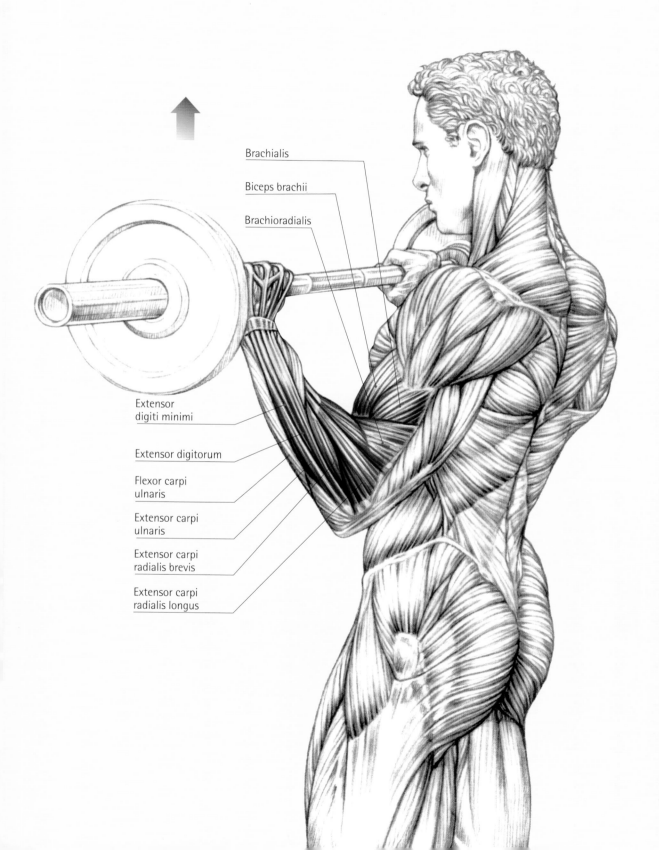

Brachialis

Biceps brachii

Brachioradialis

Extensor
digiti minimi

Extensor digitorum

Flexor carpi
ulnaris

Extensor carpi
ulnaris

Extensor carpi
radialis brevis

Extensor carpi
radialis longus

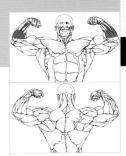

BEGINNING EXERCISES FOR THE FOREARMS

2 Wrist Curl

This is an isolation exercise for the inner part of the forearm.
Unilateral work is possible, but not necessarily desirable, so that you do not spend too much time on your workout.

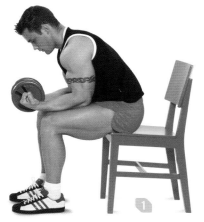

While seated, grab a bar (straight bar or EZ bar) or a dumbbell at the ends with supinated hands (thumbs toward the outside). Place your forearms on your thighs or on a bench so that your hands can move freely.

Using your forearms, lift your hands as high as possible. Hold the contraction for 1 second before slowly lowering the weight **1** **2**.

Variations

a You can do this exercise unilaterally with a dumbbell, but it is more dangerous because the wrist is more unstable. The hand can be put in a precarious spot in the lengthened phase of the exercise. To avoid this lateral twisting in your wrist, always keep your thumb a little higher than your pinky.

b You can do wrist curls while standing with the bar behind you using a pronated grip. This variation is less risky for your wrists, so you can use heavier weights.

c You can do wrist curls while standing with the bar in front of you and using a pronated or supinated grip.

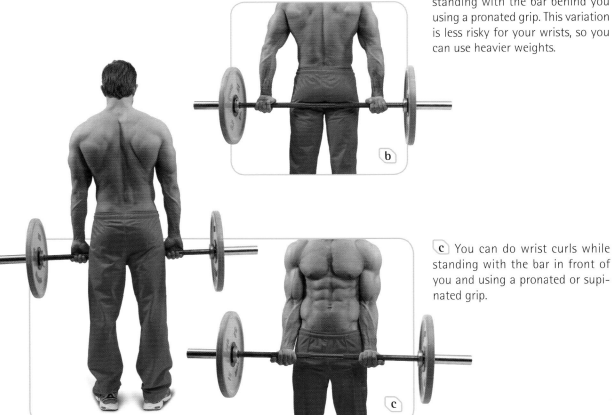

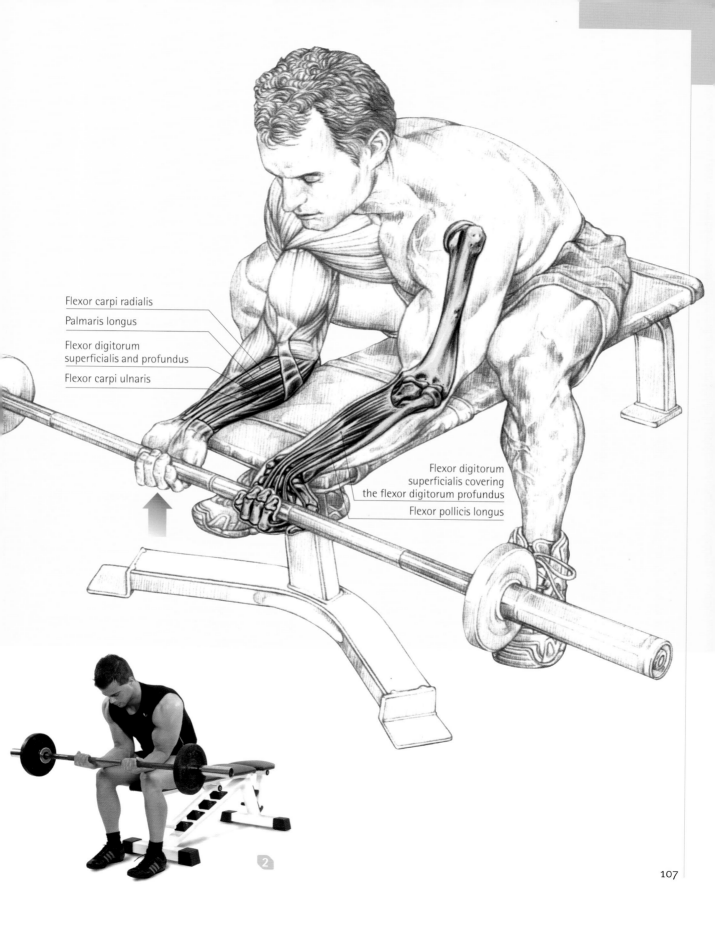

Flexor carpi radialis

Palmaris longus

Flexor digitorum
superficialis and profundus

Flexor carpi ulnaris

Flexor digitorum
superficialis covering
the flexor digitorum profundus

Flexor pollicis longus

d Keep the bar in front of your body or behind it, and instead of keeping your fist closed, open your hand a bit while your palms are perpendicular to the floor. Tighten your fists before doing a wrist curl. This more diffi-cult variation works both the deep and superficial layers of the flexor muscles.

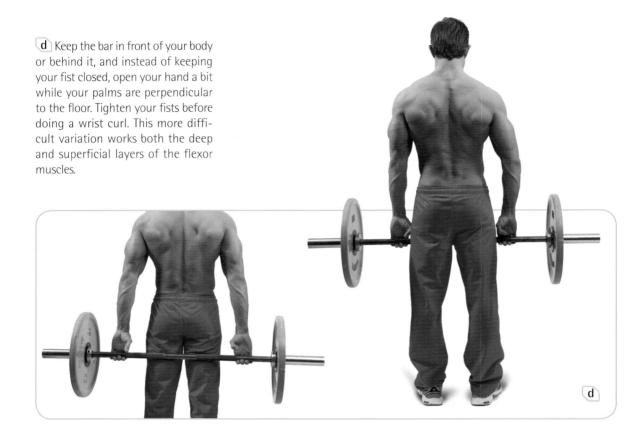

HELPFUL HINTS

The more you bend your arms, the stronger you will be during this exercise. However, this is not a power move done explosively. The forearm muscles were made to handle prolonged work. Do this exercise slowly.

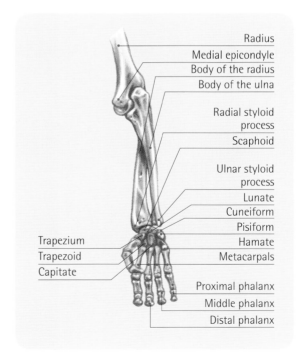

Radius
Medial epicondyle
Body of the radius
Body of the ulna
Radial styloid process
Scaphoid
Ulnar styloid process
Lunate
Cuneiform
Pisiform
Hamate
Metacarpals
Proximal phalanx
Middle phalanx
Distal phalanx
Trapezium
Trapezoid
Capitate

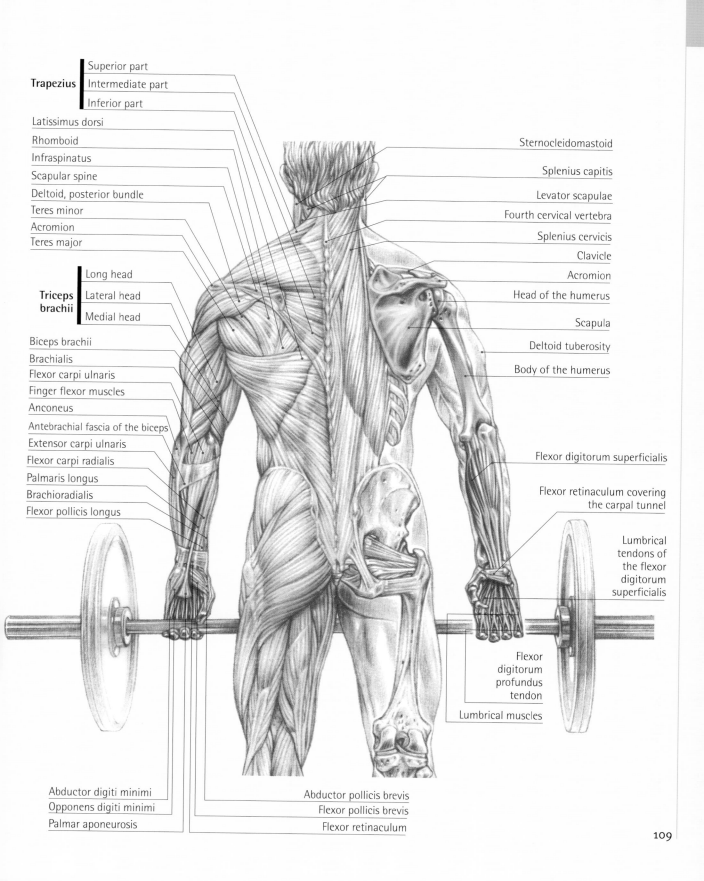

Trapezius
Superior part
Intermediate part
Inferior part

Latissimus dorsi

Rhomboid

Infraspinatus

Scapular spine

Deltoid, posterior bundle

Teres minor

Acromion

Teres major

Triceps brachii
Long head
Lateral head
Medial head

Biceps brachii

Brachialis

Flexor carpi ulnaris

Finger flexor muscles

Anconeus

Antebrachial fascia of the biceps

Extensor carpi ulnaris

Flexor carpi radialis

Palmaris longus

Brachioradialis

Flexor pollicis longus

Sternocleidomastoid

Splenius capitis

Levator scapulae

Fourth cervical vertebra

Splenius cervicis

Clavicle

Acromion

Head of the humerus

Scapula

Deltoid tuberosity

Body of the humerus

Flexor digitorum superficialis

Flexor retinaculum covering the carpal tunnel

Lumbrical tendons of the flexor digitorum superficialis

Flexor digitorum profundus tendon

Lumbrical muscles

Abductor digiti minimi

Opponens digiti minimi

Palmar aponeurosis

Abductor pollicis brevis

Flexor pollicis brevis

Flexor retinaculum

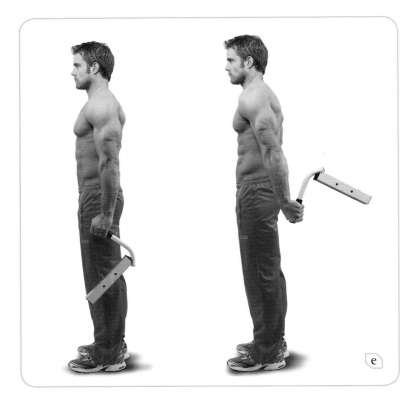

e There is another variation that you can do unilaterally with a dumbbell weighted on only one side or with a large hammer. Stand up and hold the weight a little behind you while your right arm is straight and pressed against your right side. Drop your hand so that your pinky is lower than your thumb, and then use your flexor muscles to bring your pinky higher than your thumb. Hold the contracted position for at least 1 second before lowering the weight. This adduction variation is especially good for the flexor carpi ulnaris muscle.

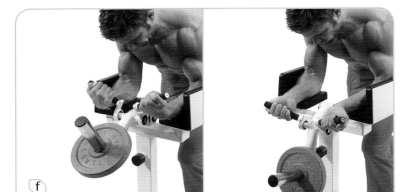

f Some machines will work the wrist flexor muscles. The advantage of these machines is that they eliminate lateral instability in the weights and allow for unilateral work. Unfortunately, the defined trajectory of these machines is not always suitable for your wrist trajectory, and this can cause problems.

ADVANTAGES

Wrist curls can give you more strength for working your biceps and triceps.

DISADVANTAGES

If you are a hyperpronator, you will have trouble using a straight bar.

For most people, wrist curls simply duplicate work already done in biceps exercises.

They are not necessary for beginners, unless your sport requires powerful flexors or you have extremely weak forearms.

RISKS

⚠ The wrists are fragile yet heavily used joints. This is why it is better to do more repetitions (15 to 50) with a light weight rather than a few repetitions with a very heavy weight.

Do not use too great a range of motion in the lengthened position.

Variation using a specific machine

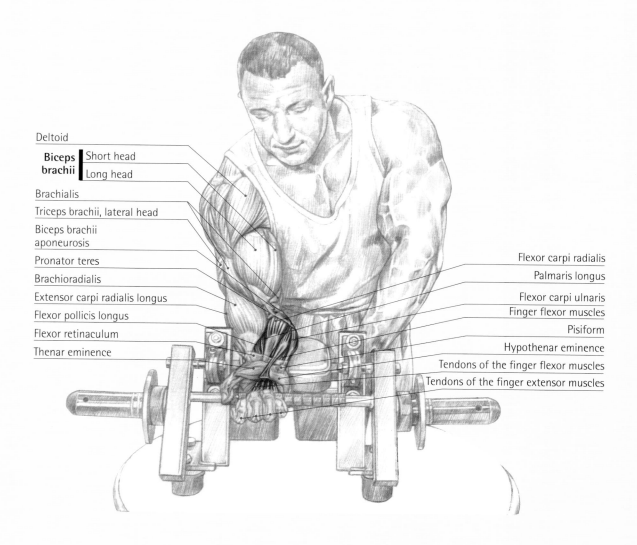

Deltoid

Biceps brachii | Short head
brachii | Long head

Brachialis

Triceps brachii, lateral head

Biceps brachii
aponeurosis

Pronator teres

Brachioradialis

Extensor carpi radialis longus

Flexor pollicis longus

Flexor retinaculum

Thenar eminence

Flexor carpi radialis

Palmaris longus

Flexor carpi ulnaris

Finger flexor muscles

Pisiform

Hypothenar eminence

Tendons of the finger flexor muscles

Tendons of the finger extensor muscles

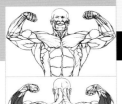

BEGINNING EXERCISES FOR THE FOREARMS
3 Wrist Extension

This is an isolation exercise for the outer part of the forearm. You can do the exercise unilaterally, but that is not necessarily the best way to do it.

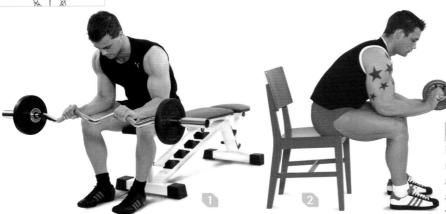

🥄 Sit down and grab a bar (straight or EZ [twisted]) or a dumbbell with your hands at either end. Use a pronated grip (thumbs facing each other). Rest your forearms on your thighs so that your hands hang free **1**.

🥄 Use your forearms to lift your hands up **2**. Hold the contraction for 1 second before slowly lowering the weight.

HELPFUL HINTS
Place your hands on the bar as naturally as possible. If you feel any pulling in your wrist, then use an EZ bar rather than a straight bar so that you can turn your thumbs slightly upward rather than have them face each other.

ADVANTAGES
Exercises for the biceps and triceps heavily recruit the flexor muscles in the wrist (the muscles used in wrist curls). However, the extensor muscles are used to a much lesser degree. Wrist extensions are a more useful exercise than wrist curls because they help balance the development of the wrist muscles.

DISADVANTAGES
Wrist extensions can be a duplicate exercise if you are already doing a lot of reverse curls.

RISKS
⚠ If you are a hypersupinator, you will have trouble holding a straight bar. Do not force your wrists by trying to imitate other people. An EZ bar will let you keep your thumbs a little higher than your pinky fingers, which will prevent twisting in your wrist.

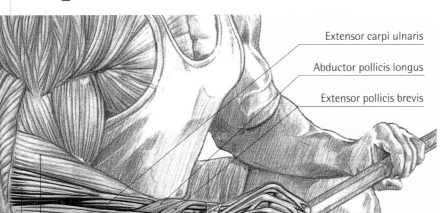

Extensor carpi ulnaris

Abductor pollicis longus

Extensor pollicis brevis

Brachioradialis

Extensor carpi radialis longus

Extensor carpi radialis brevis

Extensor pollicis longus

Flexor carpi ulnaris

Extensor digiti minimi

Extensor digitorum, superficialis

112

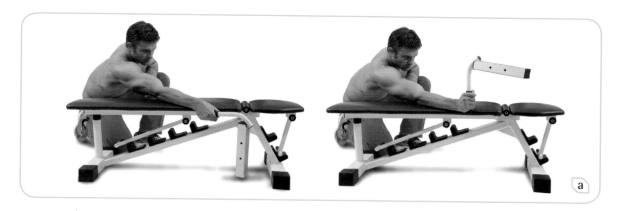

Variations

a Work unilaterally with a dumbbell weighted on only one side or a large hammer held at the end of your arm. With the weight in front of you and your arm straight, let your thumb drop lower than your pinky finger. Use your extensor muscles to bring the thumb up higher than the pinky finger. Hold the contraction for at least 1 second before lowering the weight. This variation is very good for the extensor digitorum muscle.

b There are machines you can use to target the wrist extensor muscles. They eliminate the lateral instability you have with bars or dumbbells and allow you to work unilaterally. Unfortunately, the trajectory of these machines does not always work well with the trajectory of your wrist, and this can cause problems.

TIP
Begin with your arms bent at 90 degrees. At failure, straighten your arms so that you can do a few more repetitions. The straighter your arms, the stronger you will be.

NOTE
You can use a preexhaustion superset to save time. Start with wrist curls; at failure, stand up and start reverse curls so that you can really tire out your forearms.

4 Forearm Stretch

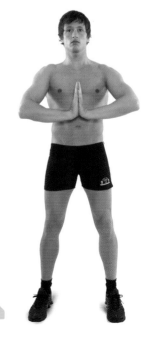

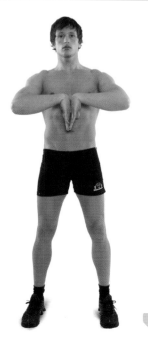

Put your hands together with your fingers either

- pointing up with the palms together to stretch the flexors **1**, or
- pointing down with the backs of the hands together to stretch the extensors **2**.

113

2

Advanced Exercises

These advanced biceps exercises require more equipment than the previous exercises. This is why you will often need to go to a gym to do them. Compared to free weights, exercises on machines or using a cable pulley are less traumatic. They are ideal if you have a little bit of pain or if you want to prevent injuries. The variety of machines available will also let you modify the way you work your muscles.

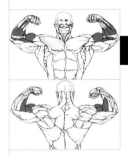

ADVANCED EXERCISES FOR THE BICEPS

1 Supinated Curl With a Machine

This exercise works the biceps as well as the brachialis and brachioradialis muscles to some degree, depending on your elbow placement. It is an isolation exercise. It can often be done unilaterally.

🖐 Grab the handles or the bar of the machine using a supinated grip. Bend your arms using your biceps.

🖐 Bring your hands as close to your shoulders as possible. Hold the contraction for 1 second as you squeeze your forearms against your biceps as tightly as you can. Slowly lower without straightening your arms too much in the lengthened position.

Variation

Using a machine, you often have the choice of working one arm or both at the same time. You will be strongest if you work one arm at a time.

ADVANTAGES

This is a good way to isolate the biceps. You cannot cheat as much as you can with a bar or dumbbells. Generally, the spine is not under as much pressure as with free weights.

DISADVANTAGES

This exercise does not exploit the length–tension relationship.

RISKS

⚠ Many machines fix the wrist and thereby limit freedom of movement. In addition to the fact that this can be uncomfortable, these types of machines promote injury.

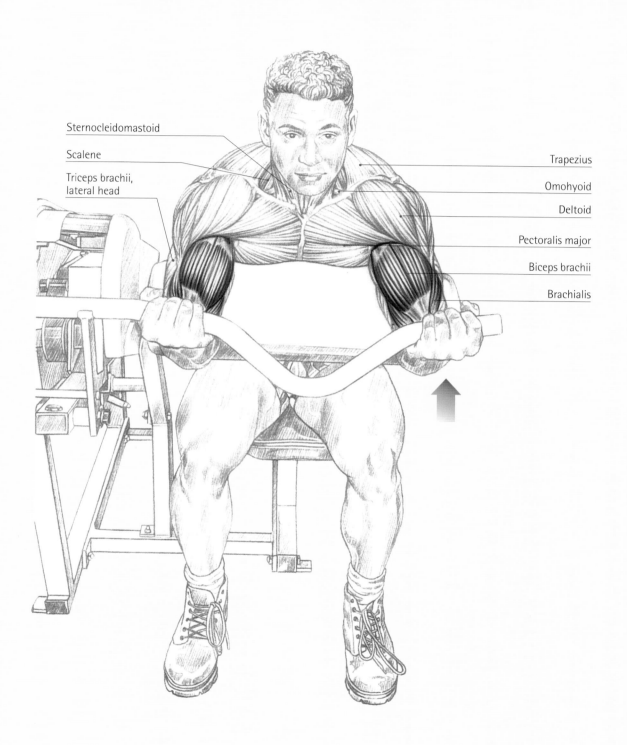

Sternocleidomastoid

Scalene

Triceps brachii, lateral head

Trapezius

Omohyoid

Deltoid

Pectoralis major

Biceps brachii

Brachialis

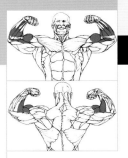

ADVANCED EXERCISES FOR THE BICEPS
2 Low-Pulley Curl

This is an exercise for the biceps, but it can also work the brachialis and the brachioradialis depending on the position of the hand. It is an isolation exercise, and you should do it unilaterally.

🔹 Face the machine and grab the bar or the handle of a low pulley using a supinated grip. Use your biceps to bend your arm.

🔹 Raise the bar as high as possible. Hold the contraction for 1 second as you squeeze your forearm against your biceps as much as you can. Slowly lower without straightening your arm too much in the lengthened position.

Variations

a When using a pulley, you can work one arm or both arms at the same time. You will be strongest if you work one arm at a time.

b With a cable, you can put your hands in a neutral position to target the brachialis and brachioradialis better.

c When using a straight or twisted (EZ) bar, you can use a reverse grip, with your hands pronated, to work the brachioradialis more intensely.

d If you lie down, there will not be as much pressure on your back; this will be beneficial if you have back problems.

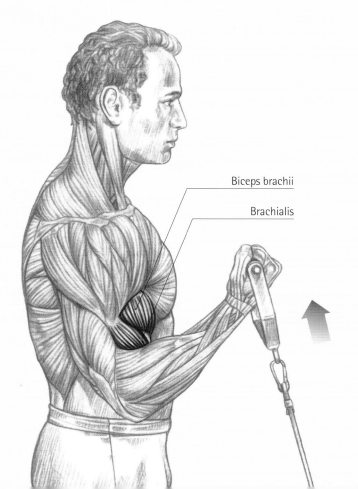

Biceps brachii

Brachialis

ADVANTAGES

The biceps is isolated effectively with good continuous tension that you do not have when you do this exercise with weights and dumbbells. The exercise is less traumatic for the joints and tendons. Compared to a straight bar, a pulley handle gives your hand a certain amount of freedom to move, which prevents injuries.

DISADVANTAGES

This exercise does not exploit the length–tension relationship.

RISKS

⚠ If you cheat too much by swinging your torso from front to back so that you can use heavier weights or do a few more repetitions, you could hurt your back. Be careful not to arch your back.

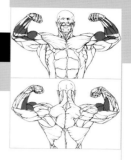

3 Cable Stretch Curl

This is an isolation exercise for the outer biceps because of the arm stretch it provides. You can do it only unilaterally.

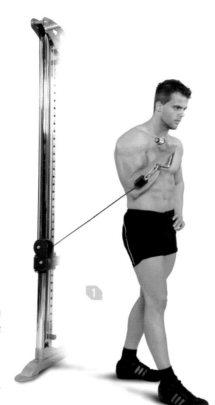

🔹 Stand with the pulley behind you and grab the handle of the machine with your right hand.

🔹 Use your biceps to bring your forearm toward your upper arm while keeping your hand in a supinated position (pinky finger toward your body). Move your elbow only slightly so you can get the best contraction possible ❶. Hold the contraction for 1 second before returning to the starting position. Once you have finished working the right arm, switch to the left arm and begin again.

HELPFUL HINTS

In this exercise, the stretching of the biceps gives you a unique and rapid burn. To take advantage of this characteristic, do at least 12 repetitions. Once you feel burn, try to maintain it for as long as possible.

TIP

On an adjustable pulley, the higher you place the handle, the more you will stretch your biceps.

Variation

To work the brachialis a bit more, you can use a hammer grip (thumb facing up) instead of a supinated grip. With a cable, start the set using a supinated grip. At failure, pivot your wrist to a neutral grip and do a few more repetitions.

ADVANTAGES

The stretch in the shoulder provided by this exercise is completely unique. By stretching the upper part of the biceps as you contract the lower part, you use the length-tension relationship more so than in other kinds of curls. This is why the exercise is so effective.

DISADVANTAGES

Because you must do this exercise unilaterally, it will take more time.

RISKS

⚠ As in all biceps exercises, you should never completely straighten your arm in the lengthened position so that you do not put your muscle in a vulnerable position where it could tear. Use strict form so that you do not stretch your shoulder too much.

117

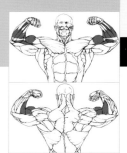

ADVANCED EXERCISES FOR THE BICEPS

4 Incline Curl

This is an isolation exercise that primarily targets the outer biceps because of the arm stretch it provides. You can do it unilaterally.

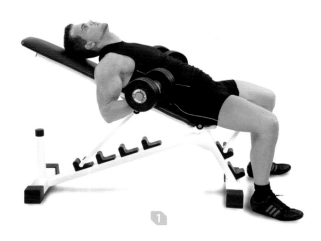

ADVANTAGES

This exercise gives you a stretch near the shoulder that is completely unique. By stretching the upper part of the biceps while contracting the lower part, you are taking better advantage of the length–tension relationship than you can with other kinds of curls. That is why this particular exercise is so effective.

DISADVANTAGES

Unusual stretching often translates into a risk of injury. Athletes with a narrow intertubercular (bicipital) groove should not use a bench that is too flat (see "Understanding Biceps Pathologies" on page 63).

RISKS

⚠ Getting onto the bench and setting down the dumbbells can be tricky at first.

You should never completely straighten your arms in the lengthened position with a supinated grip.

Use excellent form so that you do not stretch your shoulder excessively.

🔹 With dumbbells in your hands, lie on a bench inclined as flat as possible.

🔹 Use your biceps to bring your forearms to your upper arms **1**. Lift the elbows only slightly before lowering the weights.

HELPFUL HINTS

To avoid hurting yourself, never straighten your arm completely when it is supinated. This exercise stretches the biceps and provides a rapid and unique kind of burn. To use this characteristic to your advantage, you should do at least 12 repetitions. Once you feel burn in the muscle, try to maintain it for as long as possible.

(Variations)

The more vertical the bench, the less useful this exercise will be, except for preventing you from cheating. The more horizontal the bench, the more the long head of the biceps will be stretched and recruited.

a Rotate your wrist on every repetition or keep your hand supinated (see page 88).

b Use a hammer grip.

c Raise both dumbbells simultaneously or alternate arms.

d Work only one arm at a time (unilateral work). In this case, the hard part will be using your free hand to keep yourself on the bench.

NOTE

Proceed carefully by introducing this exercise for the first time at the end of a biceps workout, when the biceps are warm and already tired. Only once you are very familiar with the exercise should you use it at the beginning of a biceps workout.

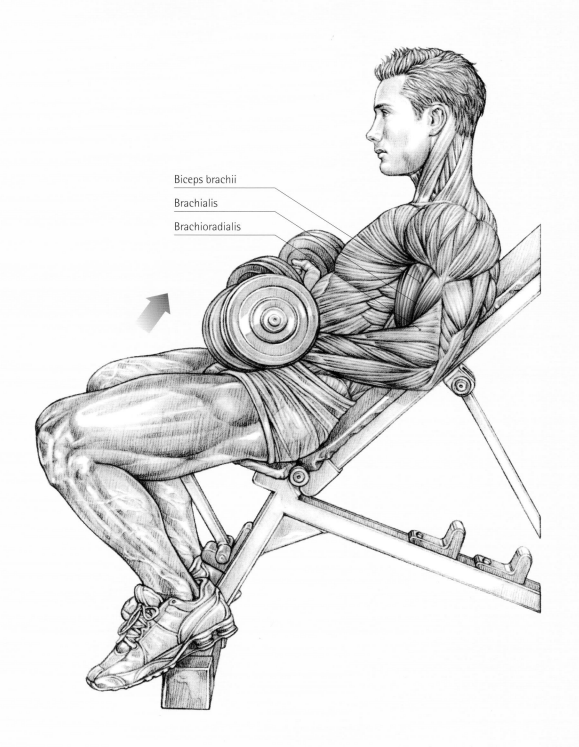

Biceps brachii

Brachialis

Brachioradialis

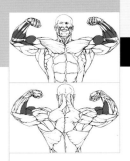

ADVANCED EXERCISES FOR THE BICEPS
5 Preacher Curl

This is an isolation exercise that targets the brachialis a little better and the biceps a little less than classic curls. It is often done unilaterally.

🔸 Sit down at a Scott curl bench and grab a bar or a dumbbell using a supinated grip (thumbs toward the outside). Put your arms on the arm cushion.

🔸 Raise the weight using your biceps and hold the contraction for 1 second. Slowly lower back to the starting position.

HELPFUL HINTS

A good Scott curl bench should be rounded and perpendicular to the floor. This is not the case for many of the benches found at a gym. A 45-degree incline is both very dangerous and counterproductive for the biceps:

- The stretch provided is not prudent.
- The start of the movement is too abrupt.
- The end of the movement lacks resistance.

These things are not a problem if you use a bench that is perpendicular to the floor.

Variations

(a) You can, however, use a bench inclined to 45 degrees if you use a low pulley. The drawbacks disappear because of the special kind of resistance you get from a cable or a machine. When using a pulley, do not use a perpendicular bench, because it will not work well.

(b) Using a neutral grip will isolate the brachialis even better.

ADVANTAGES

By moving your elbow in front of your torso, you can recruit the short head of the biceps and the brachialis better than you can in classic curls.

DISADVANTAGES

Poorly conceived benches abound, while true Scott curl benches are rare.

RISKS

⚠ If you try to do preacher curls on a bench inclined to 45 degrees, then you should never straighten your arms. Maintain continuous tension. The lengthened position can potentially damage your biceps tendon and cause pain in your forearms.

NOTE

If you do not have a bench, a pommel horse (used in gymnastics) is perfect for these curls. Actually, these were what the first bodybuilders used when doing preacher curls. The shape of good benches mimics the pommel horse's curvature and incline.

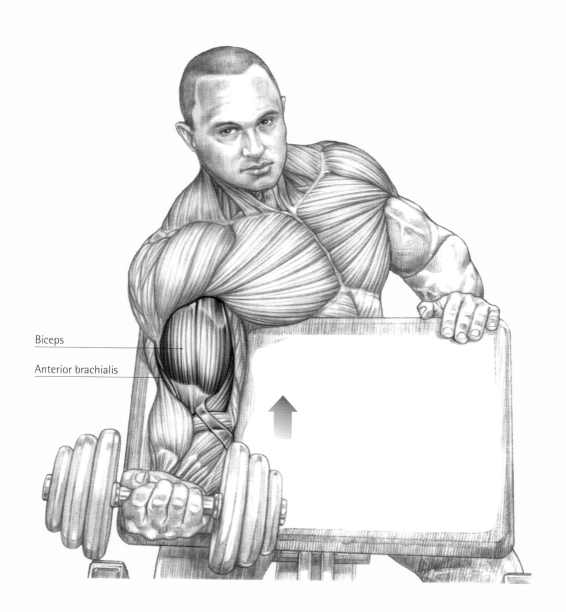

Biceps

Anterior brachialis

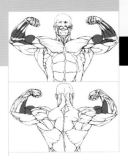

ADVANCED EXERCISES FOR THE BICEPS
6 Brachialis Curl

This is an isolation exercise for the brachialis. Sometimes the version you choose requires you to do the curls unilaterally, and this is preferable, especially if your goal is to strengthen a delayed brachialis.

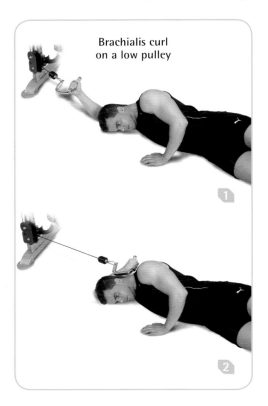

Brachialis curl on a low pulley

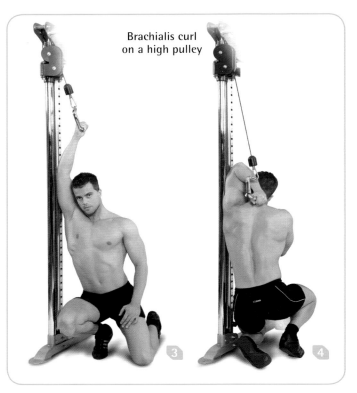

Brachialis curl on a high pulley

Brachialis Curl on a Low Pulley

🔹 Lie on the floor on your right side in line with the pulley, with your head next to the machine. Stretch your right arm toward the pulley. Your arm should not be exactly in line with your body or you could hurt your shoulder and the short head of your biceps.

🔹 Grab the pulley handle **1** and bend your arm to bring your hand to the base of your neck, behind your head **2**. Hold the contraction for 1 second before slowly returning to the starting position.

Brachialis Curl on a High Pulley

🔹 You can either kneel or stand (depending on your size) with the machine on your right side. Stretch your arm above your head to grab the handle of the high pulley **3**. Bend your arm to bring your hand to the base of your neck **4**. Hold the contraction for 1 second before slowly returning to the starting position.

HELPFUL HINTS

The higher you put your elbow above your head, the better you will isolate the brachialis from the biceps. Because the biceps is a multi-joint muscle, the more you lift your elbow, the more the long head of your biceps softens, and this prevents it from working effectively.

TIP

With your free hand, brush the ends of your fingers over your brachialis so that you can feel the contraction better.

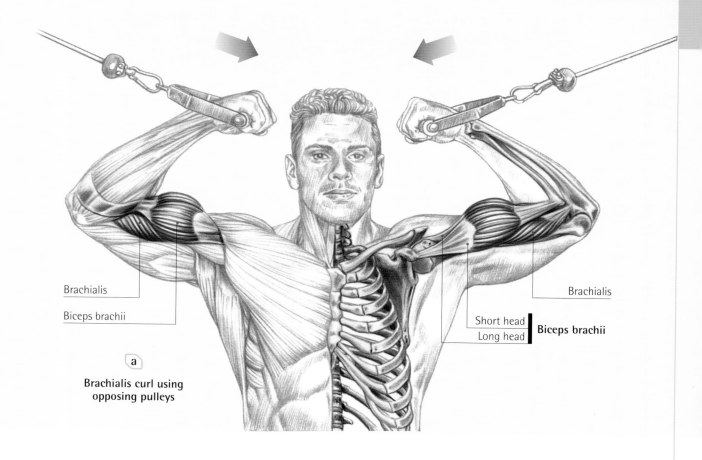

Brachialis

Biceps brachii

Brachialis

Short head
Long head **Biceps brachii**

a

Brachialis curl using opposing pulleys

Variations

a You can do this exercise while standing with your hands out to your sides using opposing pulleys. Since the elbow is at midlevel, the work is shared between the biceps and the brachialis. This position will not be satisfactory for those who have a hard time recruiting the brachialis.

b There are brachialis machines that work the forearm flexor muscles by positioning the elbow above the head. Even though these machines are in style, they are still fairly hard to find. Unfortunately, they have the same disadvantages as classic biceps machines: For someone who has a valgus or who is a hyperpronator, these machines take the forearm to a place where the hand does not necessarily want to go.

ADVANTAGES

Even though the biceps is still working, you can feel the brachialis sliding along the humerus, a sign that it is contracting powerfully.

DISADVANTAGES

Brachialis curls are not always necessary because you should have already worked this muscle with classic curls.

RISKS

⚠ Be careful not to use your shoulder to initiate the movement because the shoulder is in a vulnerable position when your arms are above your head.

123

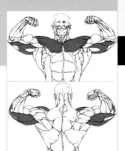

ADVANCED EXERCISES FOR THE TRICEPS

1 Narrow-Grip Bench Press

This is a compound exercise for the triceps, shoulders, and chest.
Unilateral work is difficult.

🔲 Lie on a bench made for bench presses or in a Smith machine. Your hands should be pronated and spread about clavicle-width apart.

🔲 Lower the bar to your chest and then lift it up using your triceps as much as possible.

HELPFUL HINTS

The narrower your grip and the farther out your elbows are, the more the triceps will work. If you do not feel any tingling in your wrists, then you can use a narrower grip.

If you use a wider grip, you will increase the recruitment of the chest muscles.

Variations

a You can attach bands to the bar to accentuate the work of the triceps. As you lift your arms, the resistance increases. So as you straighten your arms, the triceps starts to work harder and the chest works less.

b If you rest with the bar on your chest, the triceps will be recruited even more to compensate for part of the kinetic energy lost during this 1- or 2-second break.

c The partial narrow-grip bench press, in a Smith machine or on a bench with adjustable bar rests, consists of doing the upper phase of the exercise (close to complete extension of the arms). It targets the triceps more than the full bench press.

NOTE

At failure, instead of stopping the exercise, you can move to narrow push-ups so that you can get a few more repetitions.

ADVANTAGES

Narrow-grip bench press is one of the only triceps exercises that really takes advantage of the length-tension relationship in the long head.

DISADVANTAGES

It is not always easy to target the triceps well because the chest and shoulders work to varying degrees as well.

RISKS

⚠ Not all wrists are made to do bench presses with a very narrow grip. So that you do not hurt your wrists, use a twisted EZ bar instead of a straight bar or widen your grip.

In the lengthened phase, the tendon of the long head of the biceps is compressed as the elbow is pointed outward. This results in friction that could damage the tendon.

The smaller the degree you can extend your arm naturally, the more you will need to maintain continuous tension in the upper part of the bench press.

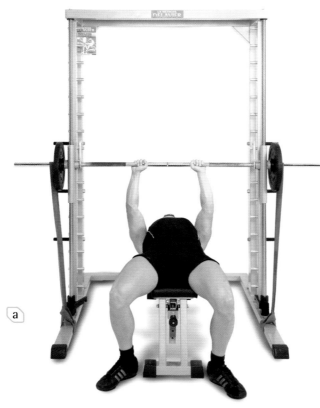

a

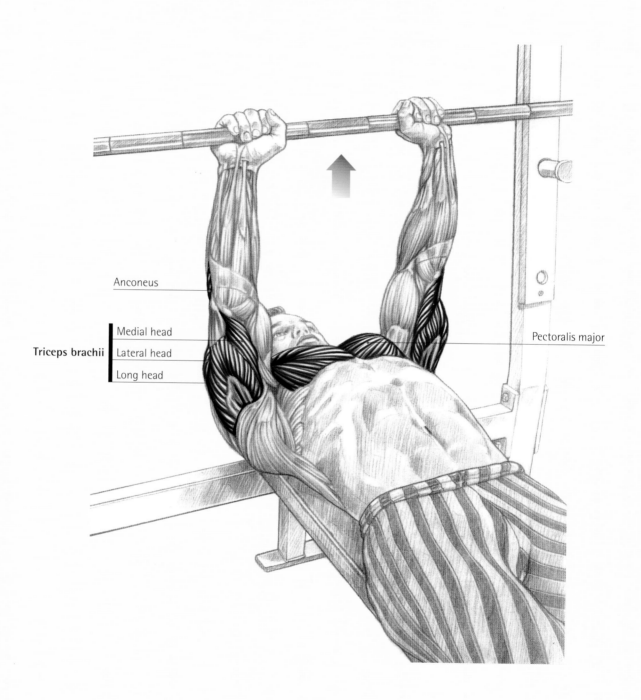

Anconeus

Triceps brachii

Medial head

Lateral head

Long head

Pectoralis major

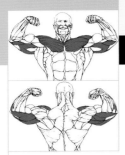

ADVANCED EXERCISES FOR THE TRICEPS

2 Dip

This is a compound exercise that targets the triceps, chest, and shoulders. You can do this unilaterally only by using a machine.

Put your hands on the parallel bars using a neutral grip (thumbs facing forward). Bend your legs behind you.

Bend your arms to lower yourself toward the floor **1**, and then lift yourself up using your triceps.

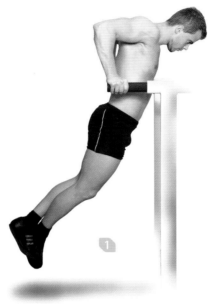

HELPFUL HINTS

The position of your head is critical. Ideally, you should keep your head high and your eyes looking slightly upward so that you can keep your torso straight. This position optimizes the recruitment of the triceps and minimizes the involvement of the chest. However, if you feel any tingling in your hands, then keep your chin tucked down toward your chest as shown here (see the inset box on page 128).

ADVANTAGES

Dips are one of the few compound exercises for the triceps.

DISADVANTAGES

It is not necessarily easy to focus solely on your triceps because your chest and shoulders also participate in the exercise.

RISKS

⚠ Be careful not to go too low too quickly because there is nothing to stop your fall. If you perform this exercise poorly, you will suffer tears in your chest muscles, pain in your elbows, or a shoulder injury.

The lower you go, the more you risk irritating the tendon on the long head of the biceps.

Variations

a If the parallel bars are big enough, you can try to use a semi-pronated grip (thumbs facing your torso). This position is harder, and the triceps works more. But it can be more traumatic for your elbows because of the large stretch in the triceps. Be cautious when trying this variation.

b Reverse dips done with the feet on a bench are much easier because they eliminate some of the weight of your legs (see page 100). If you cannot do dips well, you can do this exercise to gain strength.

c There are dip machines available that give you complete control over the degree of resistance. The problem with these machines is that, with a heavy weight, it is difficult to remain seated and you have a tendency to come out of the machine. So if you are using one of these machines, try to work unilaterally (one arm at a time).

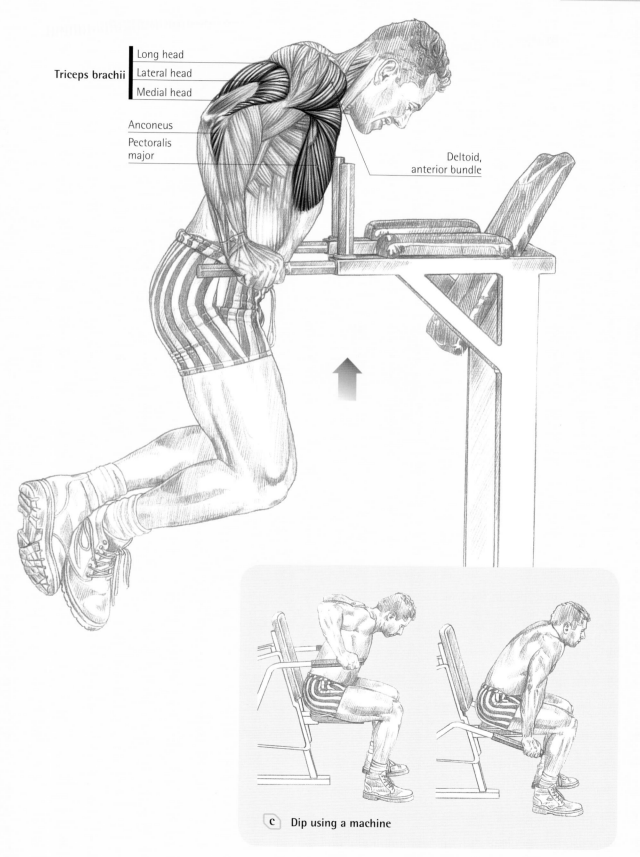

Triceps brachii
- Long head
- Lateral head
- Medial head

Anconeus

Pectoralis major

Deltoid, anterior bundle

c Dip using a machine

HOW TO AVOID TINGLING IN YOUR ARMS

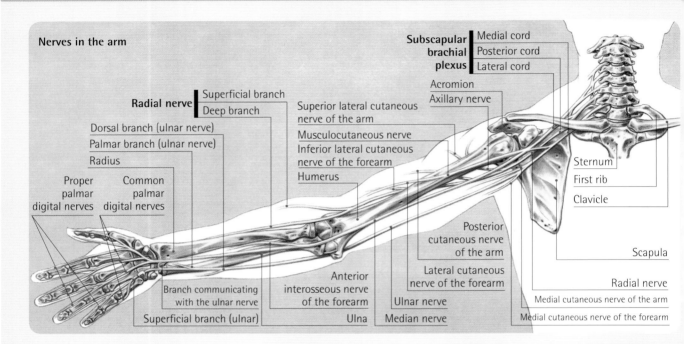

Nerves in the arm

Radial nerve
Superficial branch
Deep branch

Dorsal branch (ulnar nerve)
Palmar branch (ulnar nerve)
Radius

Proper palmar digital nerves
Common palmar digital nerves

Superficial branch (ulnar)
Branch communicating with the ulnar nerve

Anterior interosseous nerve of the forearm
Ulna

Superior lateral cutaneous nerve of the arm
Musculocutaneous nerve
Inferior lateral cutaneous nerve of the forearm
Humerus

Posterior cutaneous nerve of the arm
Lateral cutaneous nerve of the forearm
Ulnar nerve
Median nerve

Subscapular brachial plexus
Medial cord
Posterior cord
Lateral cord

Acromion
Axillary nerve

Sternum
First rib
Clavicle

Scapula

Radial nerve
Medial cutaneous nerve of the arm
Medial cutaneous nerve of the forearm

Some exercises such as dips can cause tickling, tingling, or numbness in the arms or fingers. Your head position is often the root cause of these discomforts. If you keep your head up during dips, you can interrupt the nerve impulses from the brachial plexus. Because these nerves travel along the entire arm, the sensation can affect the arm, the elbow, or the hand. To avoid disturbing your nerve impulses, normally you just have to keep your chin on your chest.

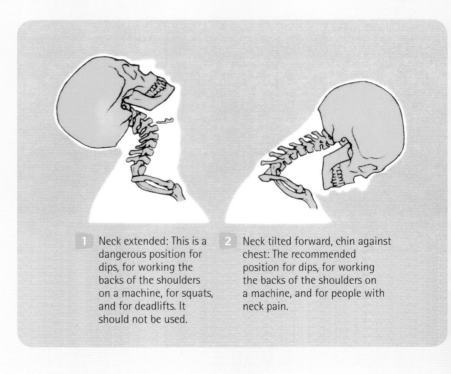

1 Neck extended: This is a dangerous position for dips, for working the backs of the shoulders on a machine, for squats, and for deadlifts. It should not be used.

2 Neck tilted forward, chin against chest: The recommended position for dips, for working the backs of the shoulders on a machine, and for people with neck pain.

UNDERSTANDING PAIN IN THE STERNUM

The sternum is not just the central bone of the rib cage. Along with the ribs, the sternum is a true mobile joint that is an essential part of breathing.

Like all joints, it can be painful, especially in young people (under age 25). In fact, until that age, there is cartilage in the sternum that may not yet be completely ossified. During push-ups, for example, you pull on your rib cage, which can slightly displace the costal cartilage. Doctors call this kind of pain costochondritis.

Comparison of a sternum that is not yet completely ossified (preadolescent) and the sternum of a young adult

1 The sternum of a preadolescent

Sternal articulations are not yet completely solid and are still somewhat mobile.

2 The sternum of a young adult

First rib cartilage

Manubrium of sternum

Manubriosternal symphysis

Body of sternum

Xiphoid process

Note: The fusion of various calcium deposits into bone occurs variably between the 16th and 25th year of life.

Sternal pain can also happen when a bar hits the rib cage too abruptly during a bench press. But pain is most often felt during dips. To prevent this, warm up your sternum using rib cage expansion breathing exercises. If the pain is persistent, then it is best to avoid any exercises that cause sternal discomfort, such as bench press, push-ups, or dips.

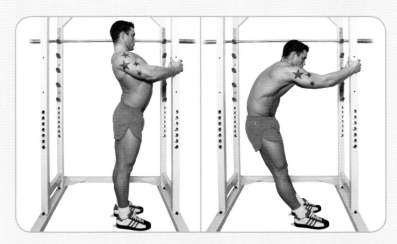

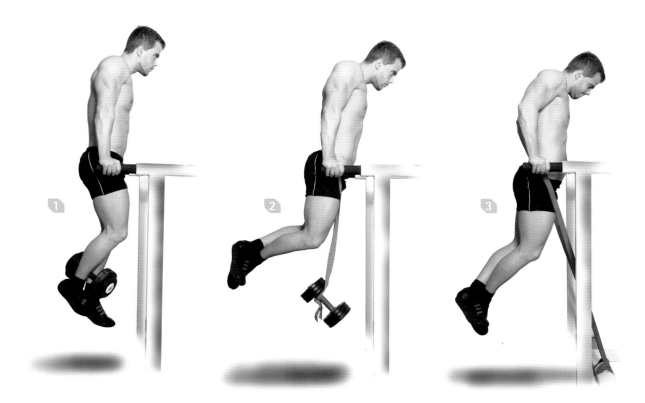

NOTES

The triceps works more at the top of the exercise than at the bottom. So do not go down too low and straighten your arms as much as you can at the top of the exercise.

Instead of stopping at failure, push with your feet on the floor or on a bench to get a few more repetitions.

If you want to increase the resistance, put a dumbbell between your calves or your thighs ❶ or hold it using a belt (such as one used for combat sports) ❷. If you attach a band to the floor and then wrap it around your waist, you can adjust the resistance in a way that is very helpful in recruiting the triceps ❸.

At failure, drop the weight so that you can get a few more repetitions.

The junction between the acromion and the clavicle forms the acromioclavicular joint. The acromioclavicular ligament holds the joint together. This joint is normally not very mobile. But during "heavy" dips done explosively, the joint can be subjected to so much pressure that it dislocates. This traumatizes the joining ligament ❶. The result is that the joint will be less stable and the ligament will be inflamed.

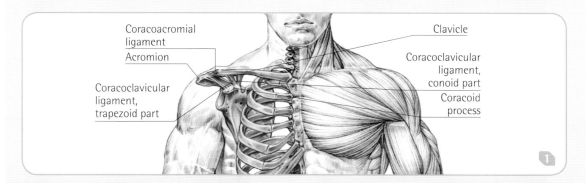

Coracoacromial ligament

Acromion

Coracoclavicular ligament, trapezoid part

Clavicle

Coracoclavicular ligament, conoid part

Coracoid process

Once damaged, the ligament will be painful at the slightest pressure pushing the arm in the direction of the ear. This is why dips, more than any other exercise, are capable of causing or revealing inflammation in the acromioclavicular ligament. In reaction to downward pushing, the shoulder lifts up, also lifting the acromion ❷. Since the acromion is not well linked to the clavicle, the ligament is stretched, causing pain. The wider the grip used in dips, the greater the pain can be. If this bothers you, try to use parallel bars that are as close together as possible. If pain persists, avoid dips; there are many other triceps exercises available that will not put pressure on the acromioclavicular joint.

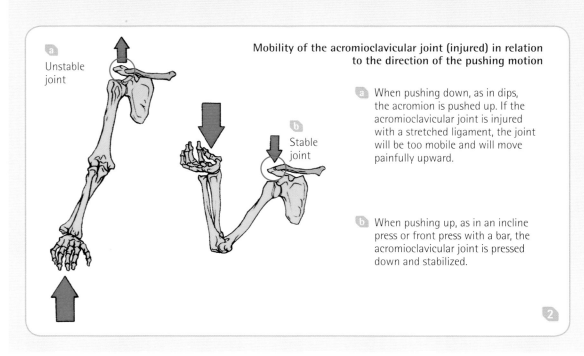

ⓐ Unstable joint

Mobility of the acromioclavicular joint (injured) in relation to the direction of the pushing motion

ⓐ When pushing down, as in dips, the acromion is pushed up. If the acromioclavicular joint is injured with a stretched ligament, the joint will be too mobile and will move painfully upward.

ⓑ Stable joint

ⓑ When pushing up, as in an incline press or front press with a bar, the acromioclavicular joint is pressed down and stabilized.

131

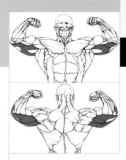

ADVANCED EXERCISES FOR THE TRICEPS

3 Lying Triceps Extension With a Bar or Machine

This is an isolation exercise for the triceps.
You can do it unilaterally on some machines.

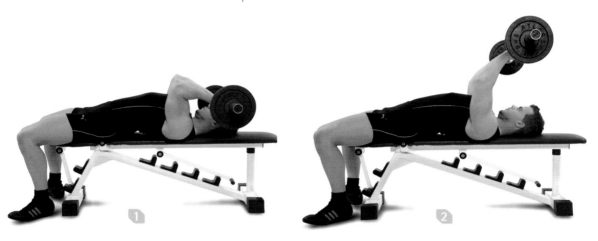

🔖 Lie on a flat bench with a bar (twisted or straight) in your hands **1**, Lift the weight above your head **2**. Your elbows and (if possible) your pinky fingers should be facing the ceiling.

🔖 Lower your hands toward your face before raising your semi-straight arms.

NOTES

To maintain continuous tension,

- do not straighten your arms completely, and
- point your elbows slightly behind you rather than up at the ceiling.

At failure, straighten your arms for a few seconds to rest your triceps so that you can get a few more repetitions.

Variations

a You can use a wide range of hand positions, from behind your head to the base of your neck. In this last position, the exercise becomes a hybrid between extensions and narrow-grip bench press. Choose your hand position first based on what feels most natural for your elbows.

b Instead of a flat bench, you can do this exercise on a slightly inclined or declined bench to change the type of resistance your triceps must overcome.

c Seated machines that put your elbows in front of your head reproduce the trajectory of extensions. Be careful because some machines are a little hard on your joints at the start of the movement.

ADVANTAGES

The back is well protected in the lying position. This means that your form will be better than when doing standing or seated extensions.

Because of the stretch, the long head will work more.

DISADVANTAGES

The elbows are worked heavily in this exercise. The stretch provided by this exercise is less than what you get when seated or standing.

Bars and machines fix the wrists and do not provide the same freedom of movement that dumbbells do.

RISKS

⚠ Be careful not to hit your head or nose with the weight, especially when fatigue decreases your control over the trajectory.

So that you do not injure your wrists and elbows, choose a twisted EZ bar or dumbbells instead of a straight bar.

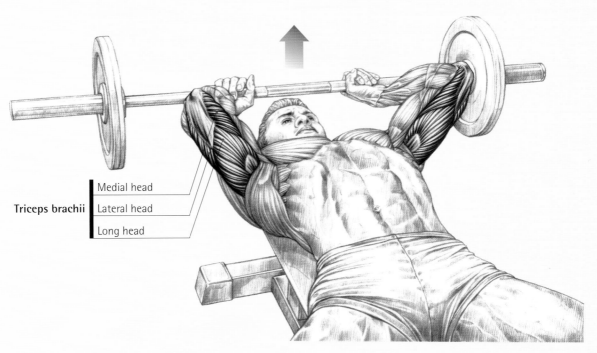

Triceps brachii
- Medial head
- Lateral head
- Long head

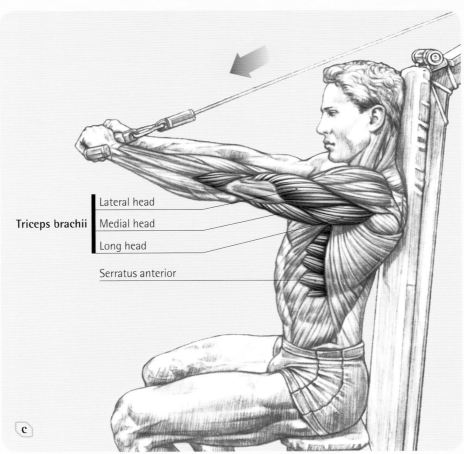

Triceps brachii
- Lateral head
- Medial head
- Long head

Serratus anterior

c

133

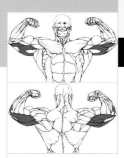

ADVANCED EXERCISES FOR THE TRICEPS

4 Seated or Standing Triceps Extension With a Bar or Machine

This is an isolation exercise for the triceps.
You can do it unilaterally with a machine.

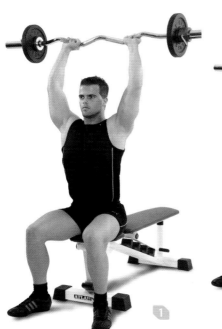

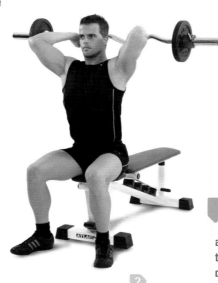

🔹 While seated or standing, grab a bar (twisted or straight) **1**. Put your hands behind your head **2**. Your elbows should be facing the ceiling as much as possible. Some people can do this perfectly and others cannot. People who have narrow shoulders will have a harder time performing this exercise.

🔹 Using your triceps, straighten your arms and then lower them.

ADVANTAGES

This exercise stretches the triceps in a unique way. This is the best exercise to use if you want to work the long head of the triceps.

DISADVANTAGES

The elbows do a lot of work. A shoulder in poor condition might have trouble handling the pressure generated during this exercise. Do this exercise in a controlled manner so you do not injure your joints.

This exercise does not exploit the length–tension relationship of the triceps.

RISKS

⚠ It is easy to lose focus and arch your back, especially when you are standing up. Although that position will certainly make you feel stronger, it will also compress your vertebrae.

Use a twisted EZ bar instead of a straight bar so that the exercise is not too rough on your wrists and elbows.

Variations

a You will be stronger when standing because it is easy to cheat. It is better to remain seated so that you can better isolate the triceps and protect your back.

b You will protect your back even more if you sit on a small bench set to 90 degrees.

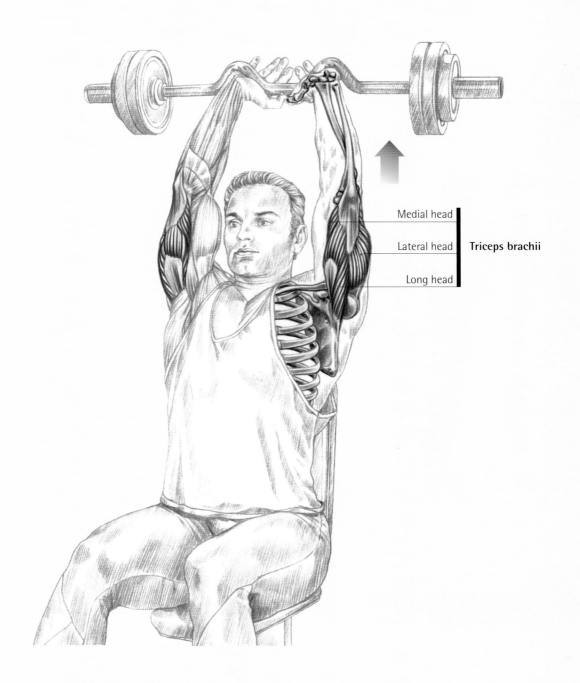

Medial head
Lateral head   **Triceps brachii**
Long head

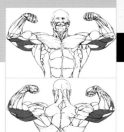

ADVANCED EXERCISES FOR THE TRICEPS
5 Cable Push-Down

This is an isolation exercise for the triceps. You can do it unilaterally.

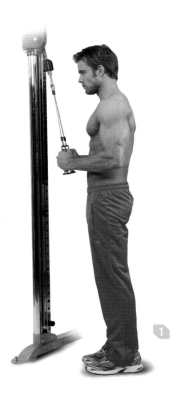

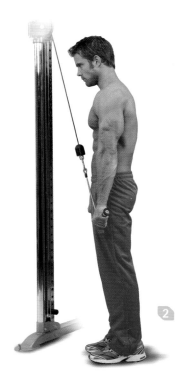

🖑 Attach a triceps bar, a cord, or a handle to a high pulley **1**.

🖑 Face the machine and push down using your triceps **2**. Hold the contraction for 1 second before returning to the starting position. Keep your upper arms at the sides of your body and do not lift your elbows during the lengthened phase of the exercise.

HELPFUL HINTS
ABOUT YOUR GRIP

Cords are very popular because of the freedom they give your wrists.

With a handle or a bar, you can use a pronated grip (thumbs facing each other) or a supinated grip.

Choose the position that gives you the best contraction in your triceps.

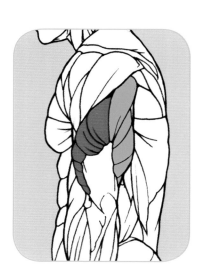

Forearm extensions using a cable or cord recruit the lateral head of the triceps intensely.

■ Muscle heavily recruited
■ Muscle recruited

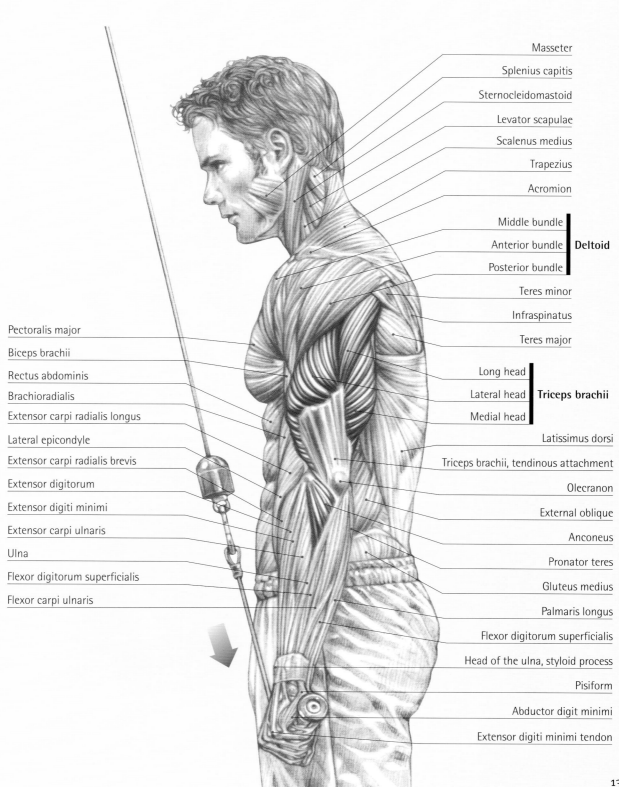

Masseter

Splenius capitis

Sternocleidomastoid

Levator scapulae

Scalenus medius

Trapezius

Acromion

Middle bundle

Anterior bundle — **Deltoid**

Posterior bundle

Teres minor

Infraspinatus

Teres major

Long head

Lateral head — **Triceps brachii**

Medial head

Latissimus dorsi

Triceps brachii, tendinous attachment

Olecranon

External oblique

Anconeus

Pronator teres

Gluteus medius

Palmaris longus

Flexor digitorum superficialis

Head of the ulna, styloid process

Pisiform

Abductor digit minimi

Extensor digiti minimi tendon

Pectoralis major

Biceps brachii

Rectus abdominis

Brachioradialis

Extensor carpi radialis longus

Lateral epicondyle

Extensor carpi radialis brevis

Extensor digitorum

Extensor digiti minimi

Extensor carpi ulnaris

Ulna

Flexor digitorum superficialis

Flexor carpi ulnaris

Variations

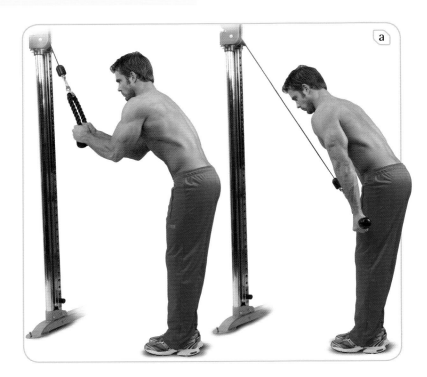

[a] Triceps–back combination: Rather than keep your arms next to your body as in the classic version, lift them parallel with your hands. Instead of the bar coming to your lower chest, it will come up to your neck. Your forearms will be almost parallel to the floor at the end of the lengthened phase. Bring the bar to waist level using the back and the triceps. This combination will let you use heavier weights and contract the long head of the triceps at both ends.

A possible combination is to begin the exercise by keeping your arms at the sides of your body. At failure, lift your elbows more and more during the lengthened phase so that your back muscles can help your triceps push the bar down.

This variation is very helpful for many sports in which you need to bring the arms toward the body (such as swimming and climbing; see "Strength Training Programs Designed for Your Sport" on page 166).

[b] Instead of facing the machine, you can turn your back to it. In this position, the triceps will get an even better stretch. However, the pressure on your elbow is great, which might be painful.

[c] Still keeping your back to the machine, lean forward with your biceps next to your head, similar to the position for lying extensions using a bar. The long head of the triceps will get more of a stretch this way.

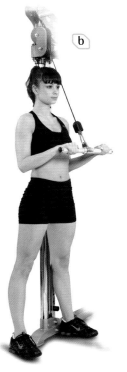

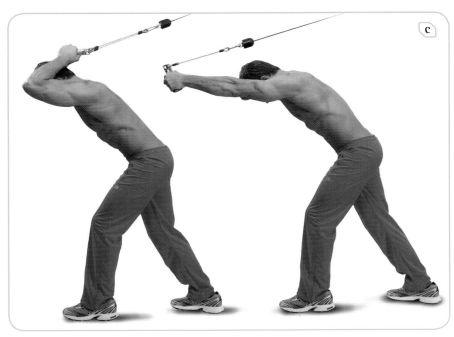

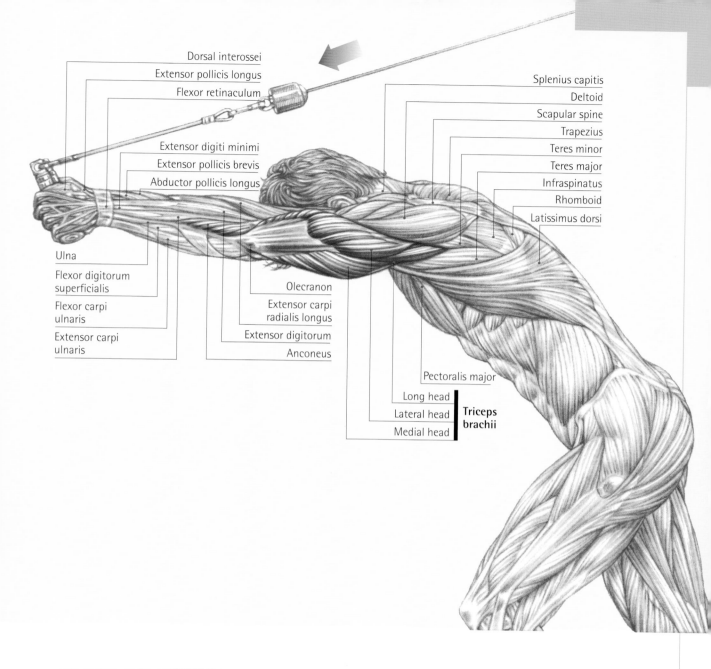

Dorsal interossei

Extensor pollicis longus

Flexor retinaculum

Extensor digiti minimi

Extensor pollicis brevis

Abductor pollicis longus

Ulna

Flexor digitorum superficialis

Flexor carpi ulnaris

Extensor carpi ulnaris

Olecranon

Extensor carpi radialis longus

Extensor digitorum

Anconeus

Splenius capitis

Deltoid

Scapular spine

Trapezius

Teres minor

Teres major

Infraspinatus

Rhomboid

Latissimus dorsi

Pectoralis major

Long head
Lateral head
Medial head

Triceps brachii

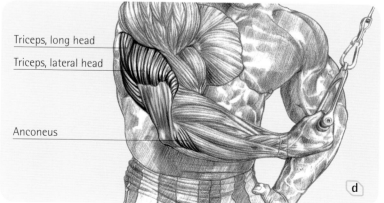

Triceps, long head

Triceps, lateral head

Anconeus

d

d Lateral push-down: With the pulley on your left side, grab the cord or handle with your right hand. Your right arm stays pressed into your side. Straighten your arm using your triceps.

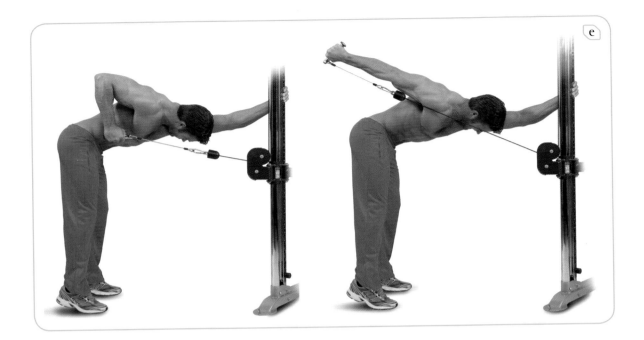

(e) Cable kickback: For maximum effectiveness, place the pulley at midlevel. Face the machine and bend 90 degrees at the waist. Grab the handle and pull using your triceps. Hold the contraction 1 to 2 seconds before returning to the starting position.

By adjusting the position of the pulley and the placement of your elbow, you can create a multitude of variations.

NOTES

The thicker the bar, the stronger you will be and the less traumatic the exercise will be on your elbows. Thin bars (1 inch, or 2.5 cm, in diameter) that you often see in gyms are not optimal. To increase the diameter, you can hold a sponge between your hand and the bar. Machines with adjustable pulleys are easier on your elbows and your muscles. Simple pulleys that lift the weight directly are still gentler than weights and dumbbells.

(f) It is possible to do kickbacks with a low pulley, but the stretch will not be as beneficial.

Compared to dumbbells, a cable increases the range of motion in the exercise to give you a better stretch, and at the same time, it is easier on the elbow.

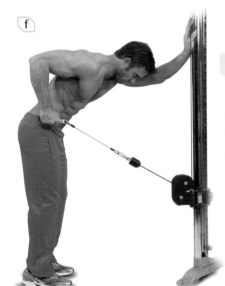

ADVANTAGES

A cable pulley is easier on your elbows than exercises that require dumbbells, a bar, or machines. A pulley also lets you perform many variations of the exercise.

DISADVANTAGES

The length–tension relationship is not used effectively when you are facing the pulley. It is better when you turn your back to the machine.

RISKS

⚠ Be careful not to arch your back too much during exercises where the pulley is behind you.

Be careful not to scratch your face because the cable is moving very close to your head.

1 Hanging From a Pull-Up Bar

This is an isolation exercise that strengthens the grip by focusing on the deep flexor muscles of the forearms. You can do it unilaterally.

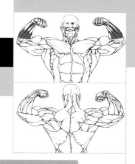

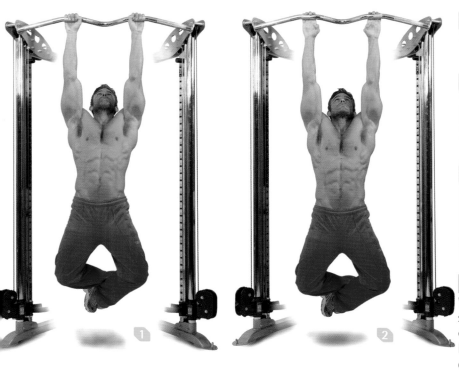

ADVANTAGES

This is an easy exercise that effectively works the hand grip.

DISADVANTAGES

Be careful not to create problems in your fingers by opening your hand too wide too suddenly.

RISKS

⚠ As you approach failure, keep your feet close to the floor to avoid a sudden fall in case you accidentally let go of the bar.

NOTE

When you no longer have the strength to open your hands, you certainly still have enough left to hang suspended from the bar for a dozen seconds with closed hands.

🖐 Hang from a pull-up bar with straight arms and a pronated grip (thumbs next to each other) **1**. Open your hands slightly but do not let go of the bar **2**.

🖐 After lowering 1 to 2 inches (2.5-5 cm), close your hands to come back up. Hold the contraction for 1 to 2 seconds before opening your hands slowly.

HELPFUL HINTS

You can vary the width of your grip on the bar as you please. Choose the position that is most comfortable for your wrists and shoulders.

Variations

a If you have trouble opening your hands, lighten your body weight by resting one or even both feet on the floor or on a chair. One possible combination is to start the exercise hanging freely. At failure, rest one or both feet on the floor to make yourself lighter and get a few more repetitions.

b When the exercise becomes too easy, do it unilaterally, hanging from only one hand. The other arm will then be used only to stabilize your body laterally.

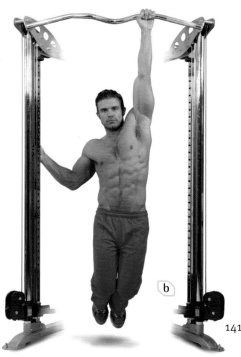

141

ADVANCED EXERCISES FOR THE FOREARMS
2 Squeezing a Hand Grip

This is an isolation exercise that strengthens the grip by targeting the deep flexor muscles of the wrist. It is most often done unilaterally.

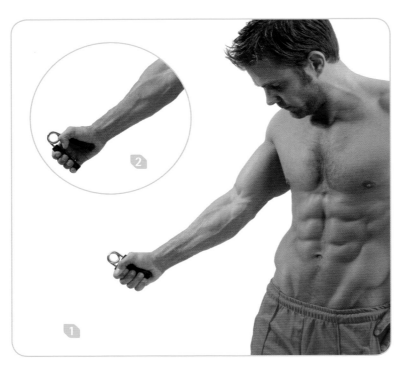

With the hand grip in your hand, squeeze your fingers closed **1**.

Hold the contraction for 1 to 2 seconds before slowly opening your hand **2**.

HELPFUL HINTS
This exercise is often done unilaterally. But if your sport requires you to squeeze both hands at the same time (such as in windsurfing and powerlifting), then you should use two hand grips simultaneously. This will faithfully reproduce the gestures used in your sport. In fact, you are not as strong when squeezing both hands at the same time.

If you stimulate only one side at a time, the workout will not improve your nervous system optimally. Out of a lack of habit, the nervous system will be ineffective when you do try to squeeze both hands at the same time.

The more your arm is held at the side of your body, the stronger you will be. You will be weakest when the arm is bent to 90 degrees or held out in front of you.

When working unilaterally, use your other hand to help you finish the exercise once you become fatigued.

NOTE
The hand grips that are currently available provide too weak a resistance. Choose competitive hand grips (easily found on the Internet).

Variations

a There are grip machines that give you more control over the resistance than hand grips do. They also give you the choice of working one hand or both hands at the same time.

b For resistance that is less traumatic, instead of a hand grip, you can use one of these devices:
- A foam or rubber ball
- Flexible plastic rings

Comparison between a human hand and a chimpanzee hand

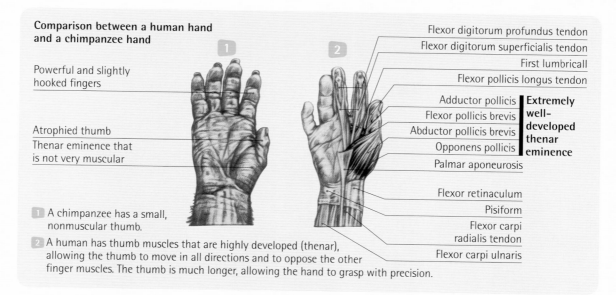

Powerful and slightly hooked fingers

Atrophied thumb
Thenar eminence that is not very muscular

Flexor digitorum profundus tendon
Flexor digitorum superficialis tendon
First lumbricall
Flexor pollicis longus tendon
Adductor pollicis
Flexor pollicis brevis
Abductor pollicis brevis
Opponens pollicis
Palmar aponeurosis
Flexor retinaculum
Pisiform
Flexor carpi radialis tendon
Flexor carpi ulnaris

Extremely well-developed thenar eminence

1 A chimpanzee has a small, nonmuscular thumb.

2 A human has thumb muscles that are highly developed (thenar), allowing the thumb to move in all directions and to oppose the other finger muscles. The thumb is much longer, allowing the hand to grasp with precision.

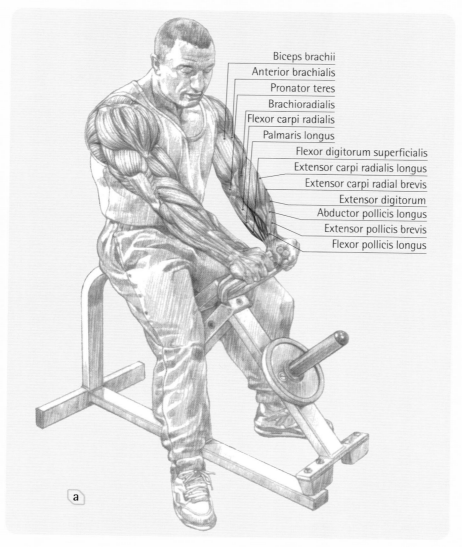

Biceps brachii
Anterior brachialis
Pronator teres
Brachioradialis
Flexor carpi radialis
Palmaris longus
Flexor digitorum superficialis
Extensor carpi radialis longus
Extensor carpi radial brevis
Extensor digitorum
Abductor pollicis longus
Extensor pollicis brevis
Flexor pollicis longus

a

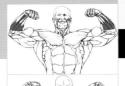

ADVANCED EXERCISES FOR THE FOREARMS
3 Wrist Roller and Power-Flexor

Wrist rollers and Power-Flexors recruit the flexor muscles or the extensor muscles. You can do these exercises unilaterally.

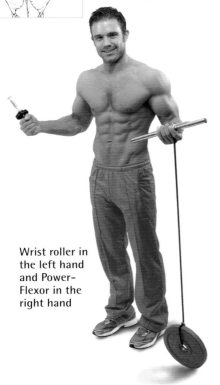

Wrist roller in the left hand and Power-Flexor in the right hand

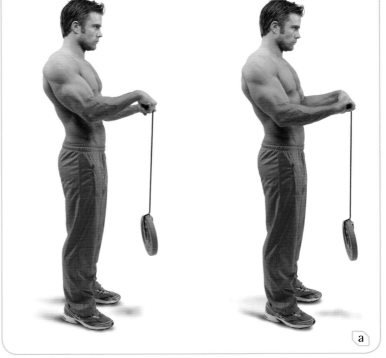

a

🍃 Hold your arms out in front of you with the wrist roller in your hands.

🍃 Lift your left fist and turn the bar clockwise one quarter of a turn. At the same time, your right hand opens slightly so that the roller can rotate.

🍃 Once you have completed the quarter turn, stop the roller with your left hand (isometrically). Your right hand, still partly open, can turn counterclockwise.

🍃 Once in place, squeeze your right hand so that it extends as you relax the grip of your left hand. These are the extensor muscles that are working.

Variations

a As you lower the right hand, turn the bar counterclockwise one quarter of a turn. Simultaneously open your left hand slightly so that the roller can rotate.

Once the quarter turn is complete, squeeze your right hand so it flexes as the left hand relaxes its grip. These are the flexor muscles working.

b Working unilaterally means that only one hand will work dynamically. The other hand is used only to stop the bar as you move your working hand back to the starting position.

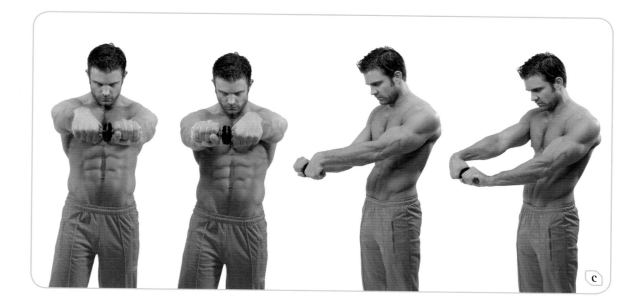

c

c A piece of equipment called the Power-Flexor copies the work done with a wrist roller. Instead of a weight, this has an adjustable central spring that provides resistance. Unlike a wrist roller, a Power-Flexor lets you work with your arms either

- in front of you without fatiguing your shoulder,
- bent, or
- at your sides.

As one forearm is flexing the wrist, the other forearm is extending the wrist.

d There are only a few machines that reproduce the work of a wrist roller.

HELPFUL HINTS

There are two complementary ways to increase the intensity:

1. Increase the weight hanging from the cord.
2. Make the cord longer and stand on a bench.

ADVANTAGES

The wrist roller is a tool that you can easily make so that you can do this exercise at home.

DISADVANTAGES

When you use a wrist roller, your shoulders may get tired more quickly than your forearms. Rolling a weight is, for the most part, positive muscle work. It is only as the cord unrolls that you have eccentric work, provided that you carefully slow the descent of the weight. This dichotomy of muscle work is not very physiological.

With the Power-Flexor, there is no negative work. However, because it does not have a cord, the cord length cannot limit the number of repetitions, as is the case with a wrist roller.

RISKS

⚠ When using a heavy weight, be careful that you do not drop the roller as your muscles become fatigued.

145

ADVANCED EXERCISES FOR THE FOREARMS
4 Pronosupination With a Bar

Pronosupination, or wrist rotation, recruits the rotator muscles in the hands. Unilateral work is basically required for maximum effectiveness.

You can do these rotations with

- a dumbbell bar weighted only on one side,
- a large hammer, or
- a bar with a 90-degree angle.

🔹 With the free end of the bar in your hand, lean on a bench and put your forearm on the bench. Your hand should hang freely, but be sure that your wrist is stabilized on the bench to prevent injuries.

🔹 Do one of the five kinds of rotations described in the following list of variations. Once you have finished a set on the right hand, switch to the left hand.

(**Variations**)

a Pronation to neutral position: The right hand is pronated while the bar points to the left. Rotate your wrist a quarter turn to move from a pronated position to neutral position. Stop the movement a few degrees before reaching neutral position and then immediately go back to the pronated position. Once you have finished a set on the right hand, switch to the left hand.

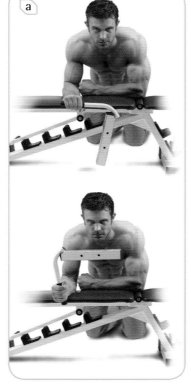

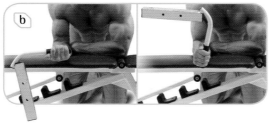

b Supination to neutral position: The right hand is supinated while the bar points to the right. Rotate your wrist a quarter turn to move from a supinated position to neutral position. Stop the movement a few degrees before reaching neutral position and then immediately go back to the supinated position.

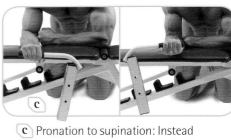

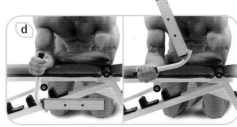

c Pronation to supination: Instead of rotating a quarter turn, do a half circle and then return to the starting position.

d Neutral position to supination: The hand is in a neutral position and the bar is hanging down. Rotate your wrist so that your thumb makes a quarter turn toward the outside. Hold the contraction for 1 second before slowly lowering the bar.

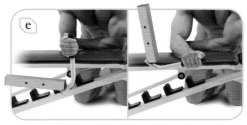

e Neutral position to pronation: The hand is in a neutral position and the bar is hanging down. Rotate your wrist so that your thumb makes a quarter turn toward the inside. Hold the contraction for 1 second before slowly lowering the bar.

Rotation of the radius around the ulna during pronosupination

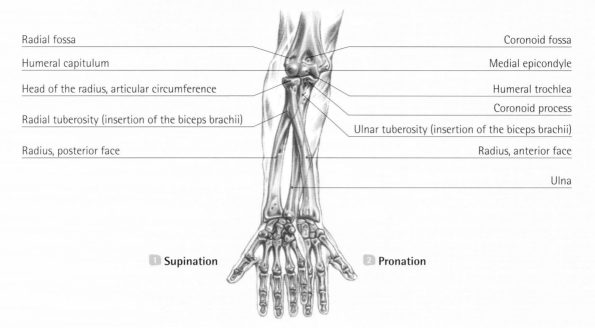

Radial fossa

Humeral capitulum

Head of the radius, articular circumference

Radial tuberosity (insertion of the biceps brachii)

Radius, posterior face

Coronoid fossa

Medial epicondyle

Humeral trochlea

Coronoid process

Ulnar tuberosity (insertion of the biceps brachii)

Radius, anterior face

Ulna

1 Supination   **2** Pronation

PRACTICAL APPLICATION OF PRONOSUPINATION: WHY DO WE TURN SCREWS FROM LEFT TO RIGHT?

Because humans are stronger in movements requiring pronosupination than in movements requiring supipronation, it is easier to turn screws from left to right for someone who is right-handed. The weakness of supipronation is obvious when it is time to unscrew something. This difference is largely because of the powerful supinator role of the biceps assisted deeply by the forearm supinator muscle. Pronation is primarily done by muscles of moderate size (such as pronator teres and pronator quadratus). Note that the brachioradialis brings the arm to the neutral position whether the hand is supinated or pronated.

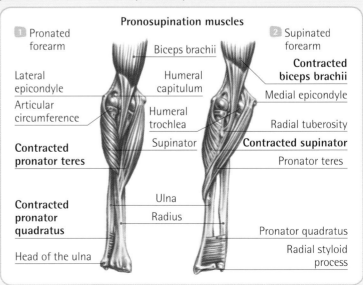

Pronosupination muscles

1 Pronated forearm

Lateral epicondyle

Articular circumference

Contracted pronator teres

Contracted pronator quadratus

Head of the ulna

Biceps brachii

Humeral capitulum

Humeral trochlea

Supinator

Ulna

Radius

2 Supinated forearm

Contracted biceps brachii

Medial epicondyle

Radial tuberosity

Contracted supinator

Pronator teres

Pronator quadratus

Radial styloid process

PART 4

Arm Workout Programs

⚠ Warning: We are only providing you with a guide. You must determine your own path and modify your workouts depending on how you feel and your own experience.

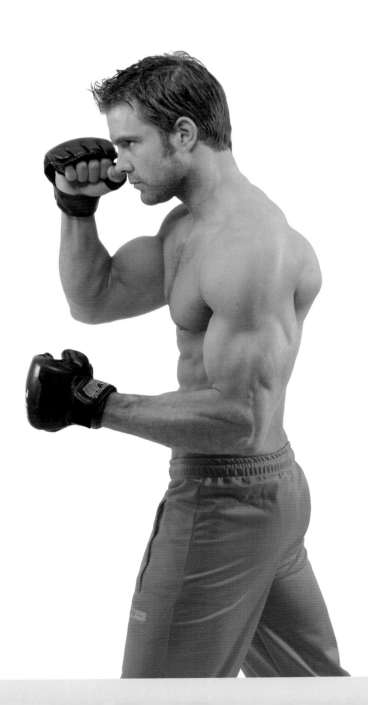

Beginner Programs

▶ When you first start strength training, do the number of sets indicated. After a few weeks, slowly increase the number of sets so you eventually reach the upper bracket.

1 day per week

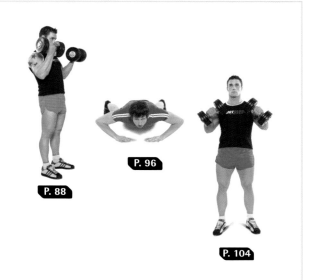

BICEPS
● Supinated curl with dumbbells   P. 88
3 to 5 sets of 12 to 8 repetitions

TRICEPS
● Narrow push-up   P. 96
Hands slightly turned in
4 or 5 sets of 12 to 8 repetitions

FOREARMS
● Reverse curl with dumbbells   P. 104
2 or 3 sets of 20 to 15 repetitions

2 days per week

DAY 1

BICEPS
● Supinated curl with dumbbells   P. 88
3 or 4 sets of 12 to 8 repetitions

TRICEPS
● Narrow push-up   P. 96
3 or 4 sets of 15 to 10 repetitions

FOREARMS
● Reverse curl with dumbbells   P. 104
2 or 3 sets of 20 to 15 repetitions

DAY 2

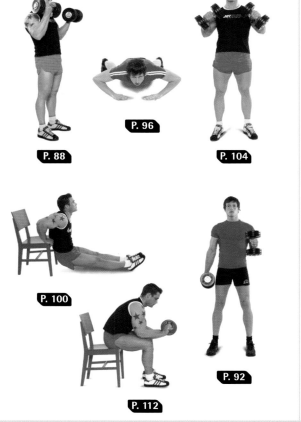

TRICEPS
● Reverse dip   P. 100
3 or 4 sets of 12 to 8 repetitions

BICEPS
● Hammer curl   P. 92
3 or 4 sets of 15 to 10 repetitions

FOREARMS
● Wrist extension   P. 112
2 or 3 sets of 20 to 15 repetitions

HOME-BASED PROGRAMS USING LITTLE EQUIPMENT

3 days per week

DAY 1

BICEPS
- Supinated curl with dumbbells   P. 88
  3 or 4 sets of 12 to 8 repetitions

TRICEPS
- Narrow push-up   P. 96
  3 or 4 sets of 15 to 10 repetitions

FOREARMS
- Reverse curl with dumbbells   P. 104
  2 or 3 sets of 20 to 15 repetitions

DAY 2

TRICEPS
- Reverse dip   P. 100
  3 or 4 sets of 10 to 8 repetitions

BICEPS
- Supinated curl with dumbbells   P. 88
  3 or 4 sets of 12 to 8 repetitions

FOREARMS
- Wrist extension   P. 112
  2 or 3 sets of 20 to 15 repetitions

DAY 3

BICEPS
- Concentration curl   P. 94
  2 or 3 sets of 12 to 10 repetitions

TRICEPS
- Lying triceps extension with dumbbells   P. 99
  2 or 3 sets of 12 to 10 repetitions

FOREARMS
- Wrist curl   P. 106
  2 or 3 sets of 20 to 15 repetitions

P. 96

P. 88

P. 104

P. 100

P. 88

P. 112

P. 94

P. 106

P. 99

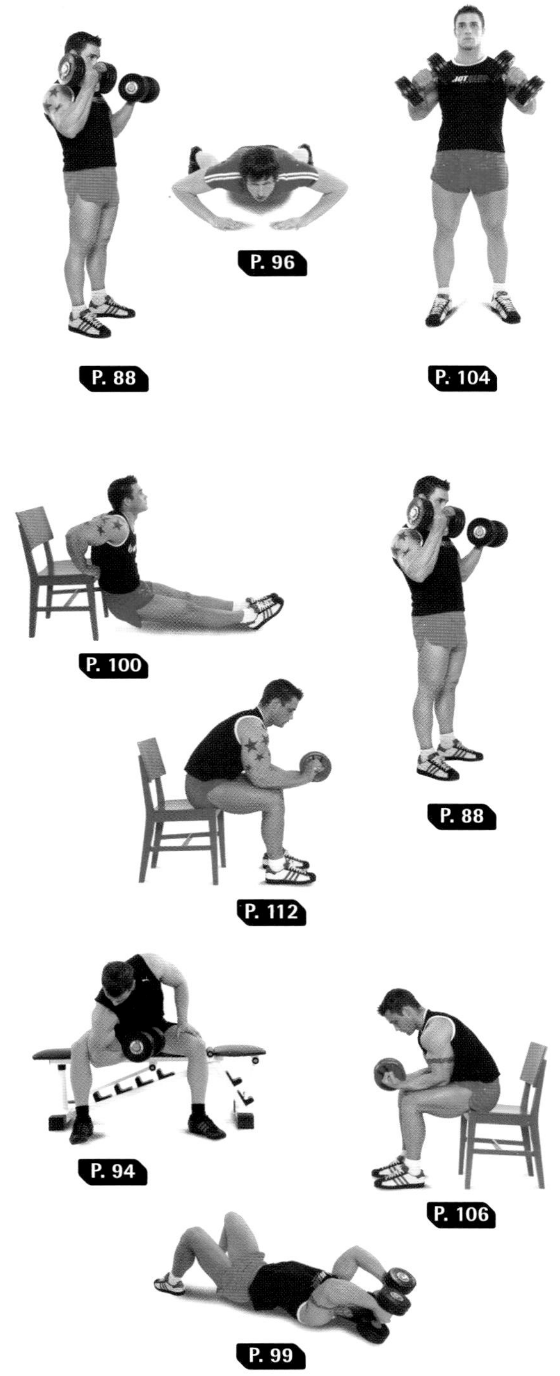

Intermediate Programs

▶ After a few weeks of doing the beginner programs, you can move on to the intermediate programs.

For push-ups, use an elastic band or raise your feet for increased resistance.

At failure, switch to classic push-ups so you can get a few more repetitions.

1 day per week

BICEPS
● Supinated curl with dumbbells   P. 88
5 or 6 sets of 12 to 6 repetitions

TRICEPS
● Narrow push-up   P. 96
5 or 6 sets of 12 to 6 repetitions

FOREARMS
● Reverse curl with dumbbells   P. 104
3 or 4 sets of 15 to 10 repetitions

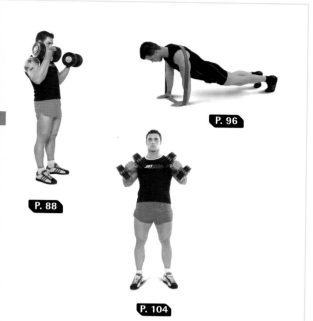

2 days per week

DAY 1

BICEPS
● Supinated curl with dumbbells   P. 88
4 or 5 sets of 12 to 6 repetitions

TRICEPS
● Narrow push-up   P. 96
4 or 5 sets of 12 to 8 repetitions

FOREARMS
● Reverse curl with dumbbells   P. 104
3 or 4 sets of 15 to 10 repetitions

DAY 2

TRICEPS
● Reverse dip   P. 100
4 or 5 sets of 10 to 6 repetitions

BICEPS
● Supinated curl with dumbbells   P. 88
4 or 5 sets of 15 to 10 repetitions

FOREARMS
● Wrist extension   P. 112
3 or 4 sets of 20 to 15 repetitions

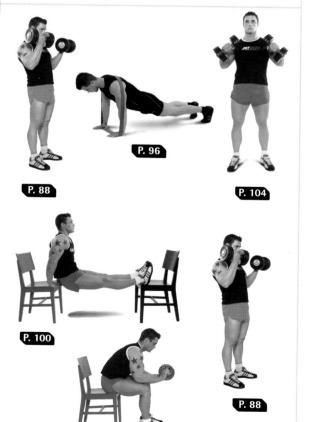

HOME-BASED PROGRAMS USING LITTLE EQUIPMENT

3 days per week

DAY 1

BICEPS
● **Supinated curl with dumbbells**   P. 88
4 or 5 sets of 12 to 6 repetitions

TRICEPS
● **Reverse dip**   P. 100
4 or 5 sets of 12 to 8 repetitions

FOREARMS
● **Reverse curl with dumbbells**   P. 104
2 or 3 sets of 15 to 10 repetitions

DAY 2

TRICEPS
● **Narrow push-up**   P. 96
4 or 5 sets of 10 to 6 repetitions

BICEPS
● **Hammer curl**   P. 92
3 to 5 sets of 15 to 10 repetitions

FOREARMS
● **Wrist extension**   P. 112
3 or 4 sets of 20 to 15 repetitions

DAY 3

BICEPS
● **Concentration curl**   P. 94
3 or 4 sets of 12 to 10 repetitions

TRICEPS
● **Lying triceps extension with dumbbells**   P. 99
3 or 4 sets of 12 to 10 repetitions

FOREARMS
● **Wrist curl**   P. 106
3 or 4 sets of 20 to 15 repetitions

P. 100

P. 88

P. 104

P. 96

P. 92

P. 112

P. 94

P. 99

P. 106

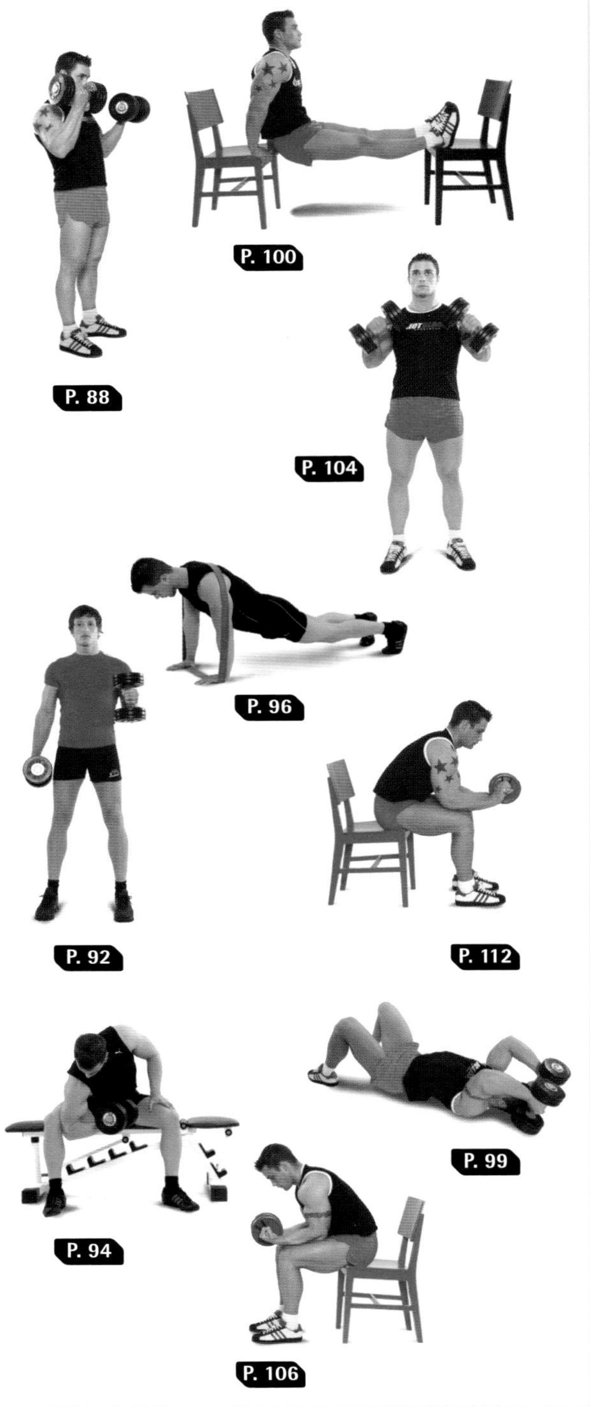

Advanced Programs

▶ After a few months of using the intermediate programs, you can move on to the advanced programs.

2 days per week

DAY 1

BICEPS
- Supinated curl with dumbbells   P. 88
  4 or 5 sets of 10 to 6 repetitions
- Concentration curl   P. 94
  2 or 3 sets of 15 to 12 repetitions

TRICEPS
- Narrow push-up   P. 96
  4 or 5 sets of 12 to 10 repetitions
- Triceps kickback   P. 102
  2 or 3 sets of 12 to 10 repetitions

DAY 2

TRICEPS
- Lying triceps extension with dumbbells   P. 99
  4 or 5 sets of 12 to 8 repetitions
- Reverse dip   P. 100
  3 or 4 sets of 12 to 10 repetitions

BICEPS
- Hammer curl   P. 92
  3 to 5 sets of 12 to 10 repetitions

FOREARMS
- Reverse curl with dumbbells   P. 104
  3 or 4 sets of 15 to 10 repetitions

3 days per week

DAY 1

BICEPS
- Supinated curl with dumbbells   P. 88
  3 or 4 sets of 10 to 6 repetitions
- Concentration curl   P. 94
  2 or 3 sets of 15 to 12 repetitions

TRICEPS
- Narrow push-up   P. 96
  3 or 4 sets of 12 to 10 repetitions
- Triceps kickback   P. 102
  2 or 3 sets of 12 to 10 repetitions

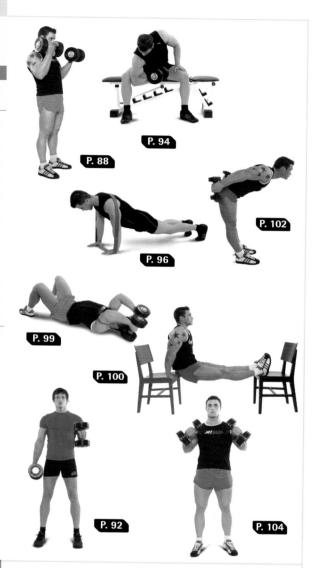

P. 94

P. 88

P. 102

P. 96

P. 99

P. 100

P. 92

P. 104

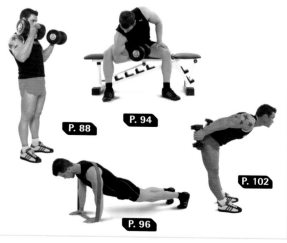

P. 88

P. 94

P. 102

P. 96

HOME-BASED PROGRAMS USING LITTLE EQUIPMENT

DAY 2

TRICEPS
- **Lying triceps extension with dumbbells**   P. 99
  2 or 3 sets of 12 to 8 repetitions
- **Reverse dip**   P. 100
  4 or 5 sets of 12 to 10 repetitions

BICEPS
- **Supinated curl with dumbbells**   P. 88
  3 to 5 sets of 12 to 10 repetitions
- **Hammer curl**   P. 92
  3 or 4 sets of 15 to 12 repetitions

DAY 3

FOREARMS
- **Reverse curl with dumbbells**   P. 104
  4 or 5 sets of 15 to 8 repetitions

BICEPS
- **Concentration curl**   P. 94
  3 or 4 sets of 12 to 10 repetitions

TRICEPS
- **Seated triceps extension with dumbbells**   P. 98
  4 or 5 sets of 12 to 10 repetitions

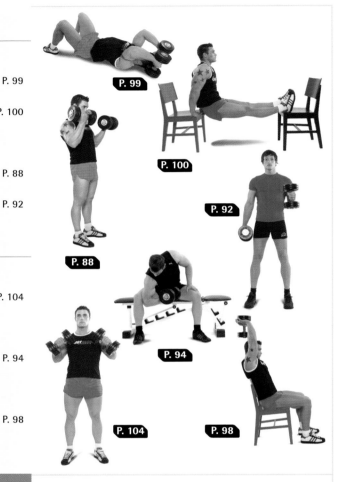

4 days per week

DAY 1

BICEPS
- **Supinated curl with dumbbells**   P. 88
  3 or 4 sets of 10 to 6 repetitions
- **Concentration curl**   P. 94
  2 or 3 sets of 15 to 12 repetitions

TRICEPS
- **Narrow push-up**   P. 96
  3 or 4 sets of 12 to 10 repetitions
- **Lying triceps extension with dumbbells**   P. 99
  2 or 3 sets of 12 to 10 repetitions

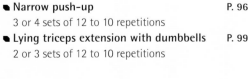
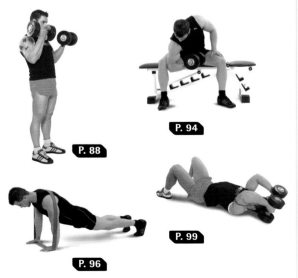

DAY 2

TRICEPS
- **Lying triceps extension with dumbbells**   P. 99
  2 or 3 sets of 12 to 8 repetitions
- **Reverse dip**   P. 100
  4 or 5 sets of 12 to 10 repetitions

BICEPS
- **Supinated curl with dumbbells**   P. 88
  3 to 5 sets of 12 to 10 repetitions
- **Hammer curl**   P. 92
  3 or 4 sets of 15 to 12 repetitions

DAY 3

FOREARMS
- **Reverse curl with dumbbells**   P. 104
  4 or 5 sets of 15 to 8 repetitions

BICEPS
- **Concentration curl**   P. 94
  3 or 4 sets of 12 to 10 repetitions

TRICEPS
- **Seated triceps extension with dumbbells**   P. 98
  4 or 5 sets of 12 to 10 repetitions

DAY 4

TRICEPS
- **Triceps kickback**   P. 102
  2 or 3 sets of 12 to 8 repetitions

BICEPS
- **Hammer curl**   P. 92
  3 or 4 sets of 15 to 12 repetitions

TRICEPS
- **Narrow push-up**   P. 96
  3 or 4 sets of 12 to 10 repetitions

BICEPS
- **Supinated curl with dumbbells**   P. 88
  3 to 5 sets of 12 to 10 repetitions

P. 99

P. 100

P. 88

P. 92

P. 104

P. 94

P. 98

P. 102

P. 92

P. 96

P. 88

157

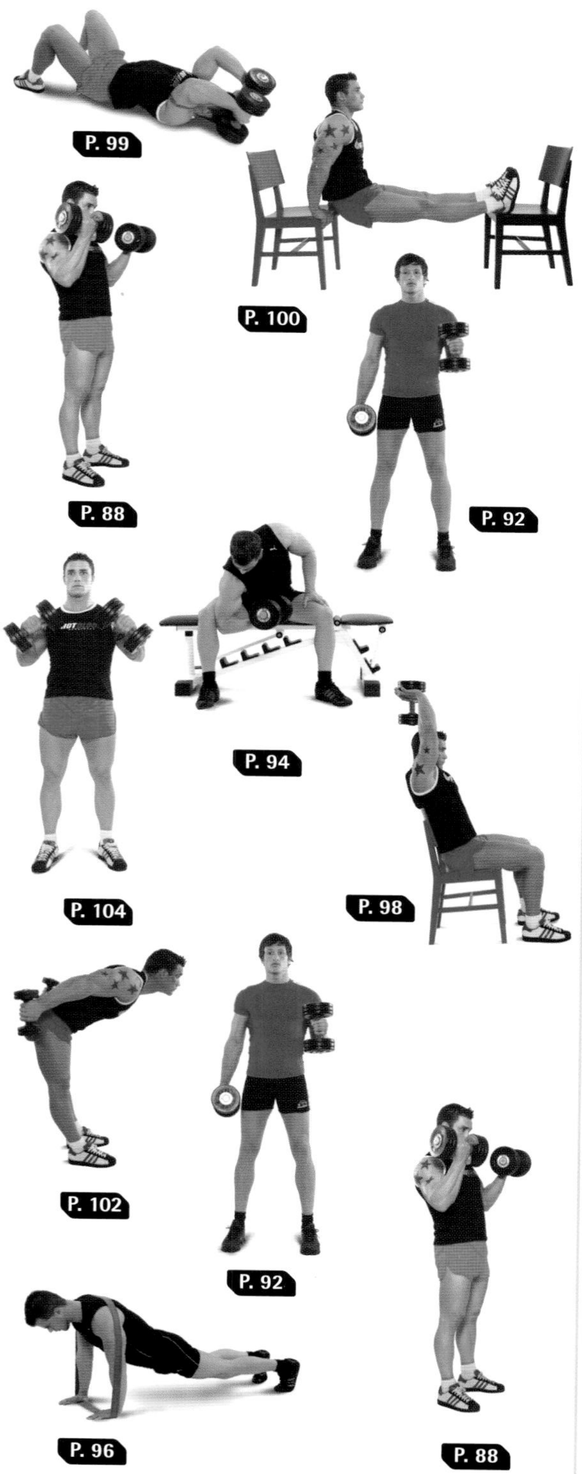

PROGRAMS FOR THE GYM

Beginner Programs

▶ Gradually increase the number of sets.

1 day per week

BICEPS
- Supinated curl with a bar — P. 88
  2 or 3 sets of 12 to 8 repetitions

TRICEPS
- Narrow-grip bench press — P. 124
  2 or 3 sets of 12 to 8 repetitions

FOREARMS
- Reverse curl with a low pulley — P. 116
  2 or 3 sets of 20 to 15 repetitions

TRICEPS
- Triceps extension with a machine — P. 132
  2 or 3 sets of 15 to 8 repetitions

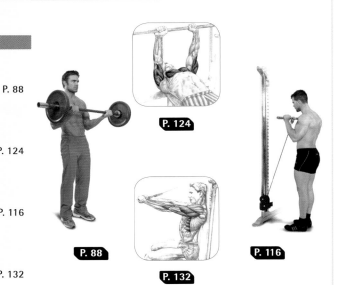

P. 124

P. 88

P. 132

P. 116

2 days per week

DAY 1

BICEPS
- Supinated curl with dumbbells — P. 88
  3 or 4 sets of 12 to 8 repetitions

TRICEPS
- Narrow-grip bench press — P. 124
  3 or 4 sets of 15 to 10 repetitions

FOREARMS
- Reverse curl — P. 104
  2 or 3 sets of 20 to 15 repetitions

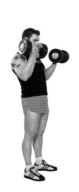

P. 124

P. 88

P. 104

DAY 2

TRICEPS
- Triceps extension with a machine — P. 132
  3 or 4 sets of 12 to 8 repetitions

BICEPS
- Supinated curl with a machine — P. 114
  3 or 4 sets of 15 to 10 repetitions

FOREARMS
- Wrist extension — P. 112
  2 or 3 sets of 20 to 15 repetitions

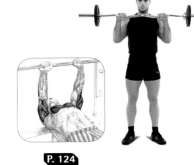

P. 132

P. 114

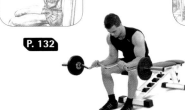

P. 112

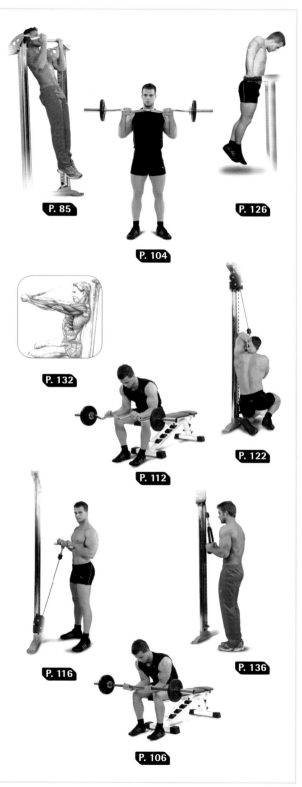

P. 85

P. 126

P. 104

P. 132

P. 112

P. 122

P. 116

P. 136

P. 106

PROGRAMS FOR THE GYM

Intermediate Programs

▶ After a few weeks of doing the beginner programs, you can move on to the intermediate programs.

Note: For pull-ups, use a narrow grip with supinated hands. As often as you can, do the exercise with additional weight.

1 day per week

BICEPS
- Supinated curl with a bar   P. 88
  3 to 5 sets of 12 to 8 repetitions
- Pull-up   P. 85
  3 or 4 sets of 12 to 8 repetitions

TRICEPS
- Narrow-grip bench press   P. 124
  4 or 5 sets of 12 to 8 repetitions
- Cable push-down   P. 136
  2 or 3 sets of 12 to 10 repetitions

FOREARMS
- Wrist extension   P. 112
  3 to 5 sets of 20 to 15 repetitions

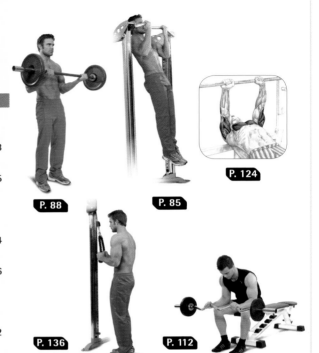

P. 88   P. 85   P. 124   P. 136   P. 112

2 days per week

DAY 1

BICEPS
- Supinated curl with a bar   P. 88
  3 to 5 sets of 12 to 8 repetitions
- Pull-up   P. 85
  3 or 4 sets of 12 to 8 repetitions

TRICEPS
- Dip   P. 126
  4 or 5 sets of 12 to 8 repetitions
- Cable push-down   P. 136
  2 or 3 sets of 12 to 10 repetitions

FOREARMS
- Wrist extension   P. 112
  3 to 5 sets of 20 to 15 repetitions

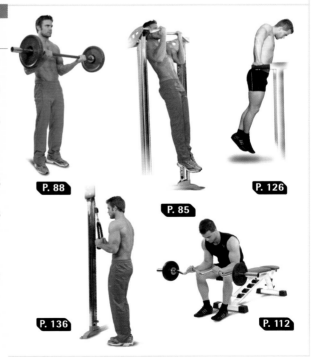

P. 88   P. 126   P. 85   P. 136   P. 112

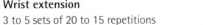

DAY 2

Triceps
- **Triceps extension with a machine**   P. 132
  3 or 4 sets of 12 to 8 repetitions
- **Cable push-down**   P. 136
  2 or 3 sets of 12 to 10 repetitions

Biceps
- **Supinated curl with a machine**   P. 114
  3 or 4 sets of 15 to 10 repetitions
- **Cable stretch curl**   P. 117
  2 or 3 sets of 12 to 10 repetitions

Forearms
- **Reverse curl with a bar**   P. 104
  2 or 3 sets of 20 to 15 repetitions

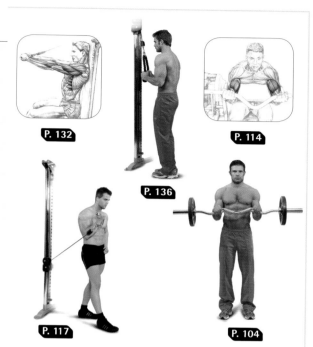

P. 132

P. 114

P. 136

P. 117

P. 104

3 days per week

DAY 1

Biceps
- **Pull-up**   P. 85
  3 or 4 sets of 12 to 8 repetitions
- **Supinated curl with a bar**   P. 88
  3 to 5 sets of 12 to 8 repetitions

Triceps
- **Cable push-down**   P. 136
  2 or 3 sets of 12 to 10 repetitions
- **Narrow-grip bench press**   P. 124
  4 or 5 sets of 12 to 8 repetitions

Forearms
- **Wrist extension**   P. 112
  3 to 5 sets of 20 to 15 repetitions

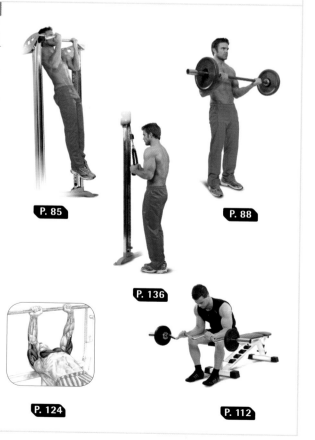

P. 85

P. 88

P. 136

P. 124

P. 112

PROGRAMS FOR THE GYM

DAY 2

TRICEPS
- **Narrow-grip bench press**   P. 124
  4 or 5 sets of 12 to 8 repetitions
- **Cable push-down**   P. 136
  2 or 3 sets of 12 to 10 repetitions

BICEPS
- **Brachialis curl**   P. 122
  3 to 5 sets of 12 to 8 repetitions

FOREARMS
- **Reverse curl with a bar**   P. 104
  3 to 5 sets of 15 to 12 repetitions

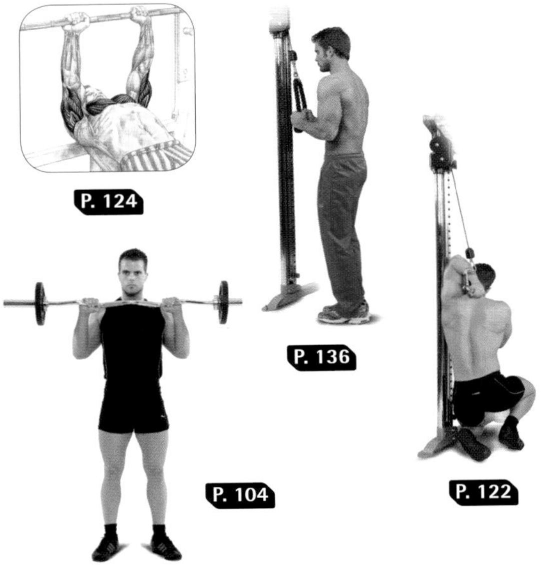

DAY 3

BICEPS
- **Preacher curl**   P. 120
  3 or 4 sets of 12 to 8 repetitions
- **Cable stretch curl**   P. 117
  2 or 3 sets of 12 to 10 repetitions

TRICEPS
- **Dip**   P. 126
  3 or 4 sets of 12 to 8 repetitions
- **Cable push-down**   P. 136
  2 or 3 sets of 12 to 10 repetitions

FOREARMS
- **Wrist curl**   P. 106
  3 or 4 sets of 20 to 15 repetitions

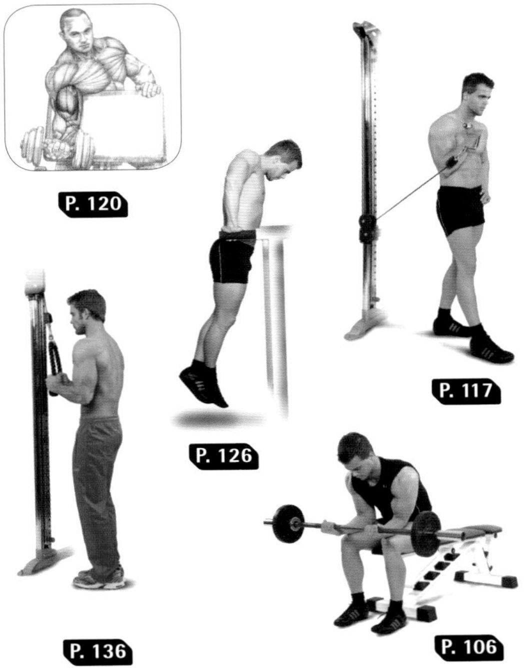

P. 124

P. 136

P. 104

P. 122

P. 120

P. 126

P. 117

P. 136

P. 106

Advanced Programs

▶ After a few months of using the intermediate programs, you can move on to the advanced programs.

2 days per week

DAY 1

BICEPS
- Incline curl — P. 118
  4 or 5 sets of 10 to 6 repetitions
- Concentration curl — P. 94
  2 or 3 sets of 15 to 12 repetitions

TRICEPS
- Narrow-grip bench press — P. 124
  4 or 5 sets of 12 to 10 repetitions
- Lying triceps extension with dumbbells — P. 99
  2 or 3 sets of 12 to 10 repetitions

DAY 2

TRICEPS
- Lying triceps extension with a bar — P. 132
  4 to 6 sets of 12 to 8 repetitions
- Dip — P. 126
  4 or 5 sets of 12 to 10 repetitions

BICEPS
- Preacher curl — P. 120
  3 to 5 sets of 12 to 10 repetitions

FOREARMS
- Reverse curl with a bar — P. 104
  3 or 4 sets of 15 to 10 repetitions

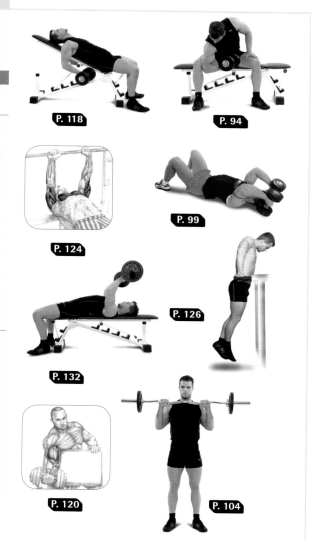

P. 118 P. 94

P. 99

P. 124

P. 126

P. 132

P. 120 P. 104

3 days per week

DAY 1

BICEPS
- Supinated curl with dumbbells — P. 88
  3 or 4 sets of 10 to 6 repetitions
- Cable stretch curl — P. 117
  2 or 3 sets of 15 to 12 repetitions

TRICEPS
- Narrow-grip bench press — P. 124
  3 or 4 sets of 12 to 10 repetitions
- Lying triceps extension with a bar — P. 132
  2 or 3 sets of 12 to 10 repetitions

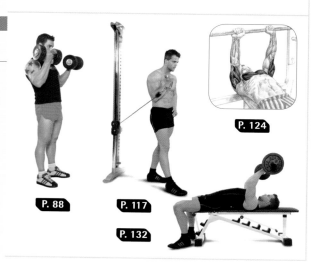

P. 124

P. 88 P. 117

P. 132

PROGRAMS FOR THE GYM

DAY 2

TRICEPS
- **Dip**   P. 126
  3 or 4 sets of 12 to 8 repetitions
- **Triceps kickback**   P. 102
  3 or 4 sets of 12 to 10 repetitions

BICEPS
- **Preacher curl**   P. 120
  3 or 4 sets of 12 to 10 repetitions
- **Hammer curl**   P. 92
  3 or 4 sets of 15 to 12 repetitions

DAY 3

BICEPS
- **Pull-up**   P. 85
  3 or 4 sets of 10 to 6 repetitions

TRICEPS
- **Triceps extension with a machine**   P. 132
  3 or 4 sets of 12 to 10 repetitions
- **Reverse dip**   P. 100
  2 or 3 sets of 15 to 25 repetitions

FOREARMS
- **Reverse curl with a bar**   P. 104
  4 or 5 sets of 15 to 8 repetitions

4 days per week

DAY 1

BICEPS
- **Supinated curl with a bar**   P. 88
  3 or 4 sets of 10 to 6 repetitions
- **Supinated curl with a machine**   P. 114
  2 or 3 sets of 15 to 12 repetitions

TRICEPS
- **Narrow-grip bench press**   P. 124
  3 or 4 sets of 12 to 10 repetitions
- **Seated triceps extension with dumbbells**   P. 98
  2 or 3 sets of 12 to 10 repetitions

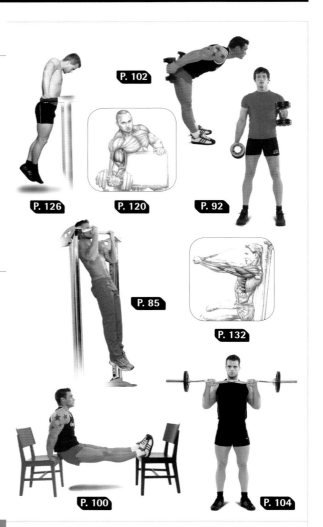

P. 102 · P. 126 · P. 120 · P. 92 · P. 85 · P. 132 · P. 100 · P. 104

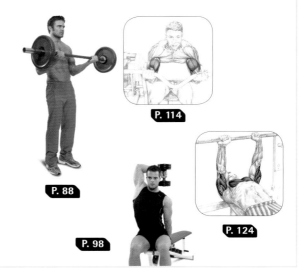

P. 114 · P. 88 · P. 98 · P. 124

DAY 2

TRICEPS
- Dip   P. 126
  2 or 3 sets of 12 to 8 repetitions
- Cable push-down   P. 136
  5 or 6 sets of 12 to 10 repetitions

BICEPS
- Preacher curl   P. 120
  3 to 5 sets of 12 to 10 repetitions
- Low-pulley curl   P. 116
  3 or 4 sets of 15 to 12 repetitions

DAY 3

FOREARMS
- Reverse curl with a bar   P. 104
  4 or 5 sets of 15 to 8 repetitions

BICEPS
- Brachialis curl   P. 122
  3 or 4 sets of 12 to 10 repetitions

TRICEPS
- Triceps extension with a machine   P. 132
  3 or 4 sets of 12 to 10 repetitions
- Reverse dip   P. 100
  2 or 3 sets of 15 to 25 repetitions

DAY 4

TRICEPS
- Lying triceps extension with a bar   P. 132
  2 or 3 sets of 12 to 8 repetitions

BICEPS
- Narrow-grip pull-up   P. 85
  3 or 4 sets of 15 to 12 repetitions

TRICEPS
- Dip   P. 126
  3 or 4 sets of 12 to 10 repetitions

BICEPS
- Supinated curl with dumbbells   P. 88
  3 to 5 sets of 12 to 10 repetitions

P. 126

P. 136

P. 116

P. 120

P. 104

P. 122

P. 132

P. 100

P. 132

P. 85

P. 126

P. 88

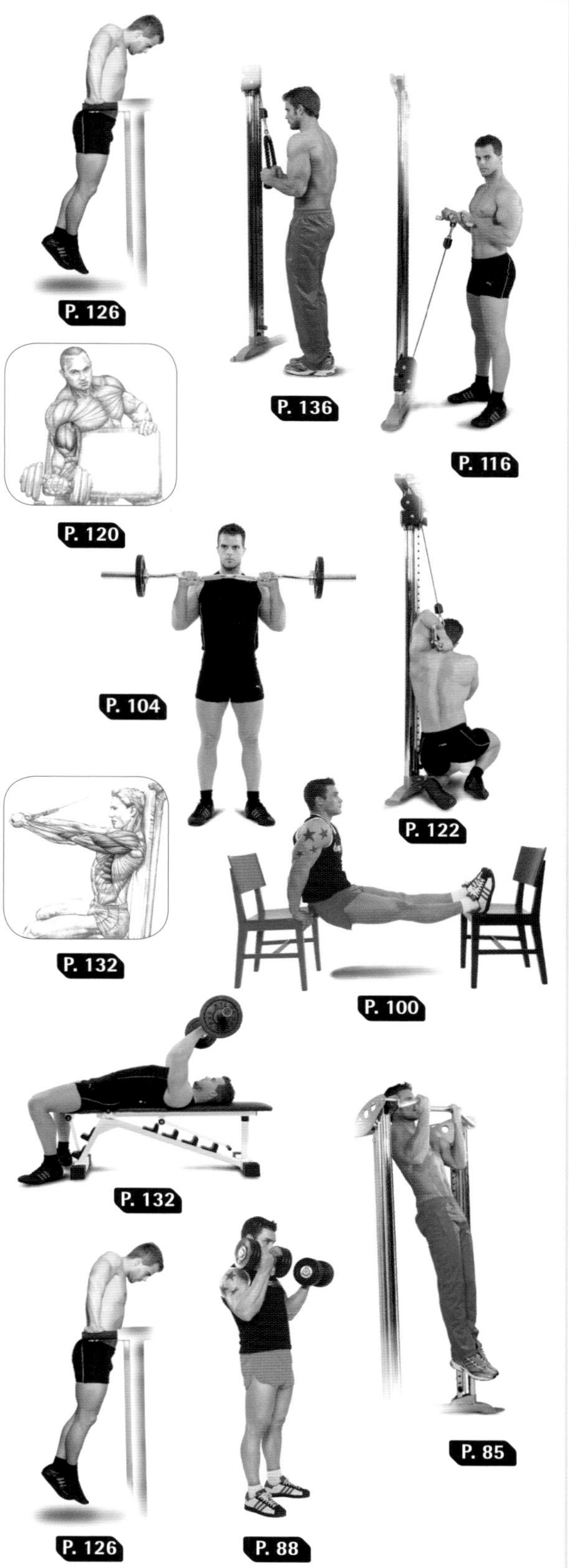

STRENGTH TRAINING PROGRAMS DESIGNED FOR YOUR SPORT

In the following programs, if you are new to strength training, you should choose the lowest number of circuits or sets indicated. After a few weeks of training, you can increase the number of circuits or sets so that you eventually reach the upper limit.

Racket Sports

Here are the main goals of this circuit:
- Prevent tennis elbow.
- Strengthen the wrist.
- Make the arms more powerful.

Repeat 1 or 2 times per week.

Do this circuit 2 or 3 times in a row without taking any rest breaks between sets.

- Wrist curl   P. 106
  20 to 15 repetitions
- Wrist extension   P. 112
  30 to 20 repetitions
- Reverse curl with a bar   P. 104
  20 to 10 repetitions
- Cable push-down   P. 136
  20 to 15 repetitions

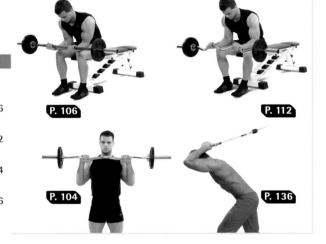

Rugby, Football, and Team Contact Sports

Here are the main goals of this circuit:
- Develop power in the triceps so you can push your opponents away.
- Develop strength in the wrists.
- Develop strength in the fingers so that you can grip the ball firmly.

Repeat 2 times per week.

Between sets, take 2 minutes to rest, except for the giant final set, which you should do with no rest breaks.

- Dip   P. 126
  3 or 4 sets of 12 to 8 repetitions
- Narrow-grip bench press   P. 124
  3 or 4 sets of 10 to 6 repetitions

End your workout with 2 or 3 giant sets and no rest breaks between sets:

- Hanging from a pull-up bar   P. 141
  2 or 3 sets of 30 to 20 repetitions
- Standing wrist curl   P. 106
  20 to 15 repetitions
- Wrist extension   P. 112
  30 to 20 repetitions

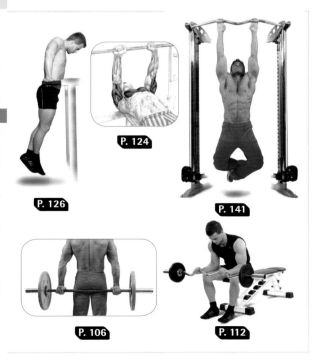

Basketball, Volleyball, and Handball

Here are the main goals of this circuit:
– Develop strength in the fingers so that you can grip the ball well.
– Develop the forearm flexors.
– Develop the triceps so that you will have more power when hitting or throwing the ball.

Repeat 1 or 2 times per week.

Do this circuit 2 or 3 times in a row with no rest breaks between sets.

● **Triceps–back combo with a high pulley**   P. 138
   15 to 8 repetitions
● **Standing wrist curl**   P. 106
   30 to 20 repetitions
● **Hanging from a pull-up bar**   P. 141
   30 to 20 repetitions

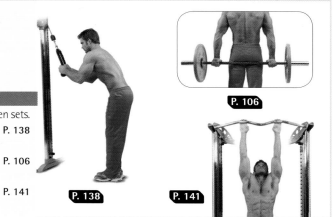

P. 106

P. 138   P. 141

Downhill Skiing

Here are the main goals of this circuit:
– Increase the power of the triceps so that you can use poles effectively.
– Increase the endurance in your fingers so that you can grip your poles well.

Repeat 1 or 2 times per week.

Do this circuit 2 or 3 times in a row with no rest breaks between sets.

● **Triceps–back combo with a high pulley**   P. 138
   15 to 8 repetitions
● **Dip**   P. 126
   12 to 8 repetitions
● **Squeezing a hand grip**   P. 142
   50 to 20 repetitions

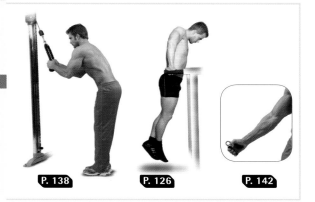

P. 138   P. 126   P. 142

Combat Sports

Here are the main goals of this circuit:
– Develop strength in the biceps to pull opponents toward you.
– Develop strength in the triceps to push opponents away.
– Develop strength in the wrists so that you can strike effective blows.
– Develop strength in the hands so that you can solidly grip an opponent or his kimono.

Repeat 2 times per week.

Between sets, take 2 minutes to rest, except for the final superset, during which you should take no rest breaks.

● **Weighted pull-up**   P. 85
   3 or 4 sets of 10 to 8 repetitions
● **Narrow-grip bench press**   P. 124
   3 or 4 sets of 10 to 6 repetitions
● **Dip**   P. 126
   3 or 4 sets of 12 to 8 repetitions
   End the workout with 2 or 3 supersets:
● **Standing wrist curl**   P. 106
   20 to 15 repetitions
● **Wrist extension**   P. 112
   30 to 20 repetitions

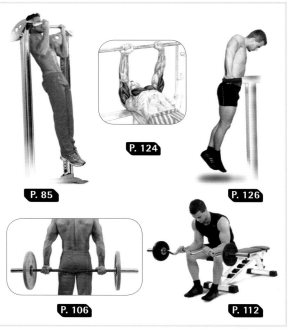

P. 124

P. 85   P. 126

P. 106   P. 112

Track and Field Throwing Events

Here are the main goals of this circuit:
– Strengthen the triceps to throw the ball.
– Strengthen the biceps to throw the javelin.
– Strengthen the forearms to throw the hammer.
– Strengthen the wrist so you can effectively throw any object.

Shot Put

Repeat 2 or 3 times per week.

Between sets, take 2 minutes to rest, except for the final superset, during which you should take no rest breaks.

- **Narrow-grip bench press** P. 124
  3 or 4 sets of 10 to 6 repetitions
- **Dip** P. 126
  3 or 4 sets of 12 to 8 repetitions

  End the workout with 2 or 3 supersets:
- **Standing wrist curl** P. 106
  2 or 3 sets of 30 to 20 repetitions
- **Wrist extension** P. 112
  2 or 3 sets of 30 to 20 repetitions

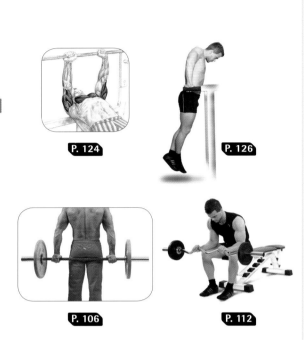

P. 124 P. 126

P. 106 P. 112

Javelin Throw

Repeat 2 times per week.

Between sets of pull-ups, take 2 minutes to rest. The final superset should be done without any rest breaks.

- **Weighted pull-up** P. 85
  5 or 6 sets of 10 to 6 repetitions

  End the workout with 2 or 3 supersets of 30 to 20 repetitions per set:
- **Standing wrist curl** P. 106
- **Wrist extension** P. 112

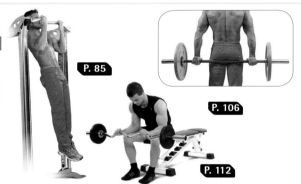

P. 85 P. 106 P. 112

Hammer Throw

Repeat 2 or 3 times per week.

Between sets, take 2 minutes to rest.

- **Weighted pull-up** P. 85
  2 or 3 sets of 8 to 4 repetitions
- **Hammer curl** P. 92
  3 or 4 sets of 15 to 10 repetitions
- **Hanging from a pull-up bar with weight** P. 141
  2 or 3 sets of 10 to 6 repetitions

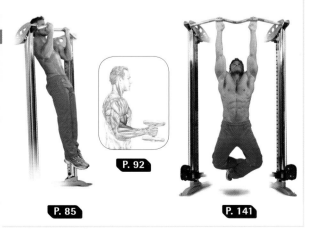

P. 85 P. 92 P. 141

Swimming

Here are the main goals of this circuit:
- Strengthen the long head of the triceps, which brings the arm toward the body in the four main strokes of swimming.
- Strengthen the hands and make them more powerful.
- Develop the forearm flexors.

Repeat at least 2 times per week.

Take 2 minutes to rest between sets, except for the final superset, during which you should take no rest breaks.

- Pull-up   P. 85
  2 or 3 sets of 30 to 15 repetitions
- Triceps–back combo with a high pulley   P. 138
  2 or 3 sets of 50 to 30 repetitions
  End your workout with 2 or 3 supersets:
- Wrist curl   P. 106
  30 to 20 repetitions
- Wrist extension   P. 112
  50 to 30 repetitions

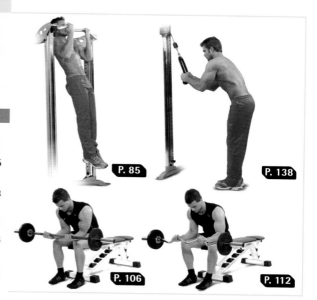

Golf

The main goal of this circuit is to prevent golfer's elbow.

Repeat up to 3 times per week.

Do 2 or 3 supersets of 30 to 20 repetitions in a row without any rest breaks.

- Wrist curl   P. 106
- Wrist extension   P. 112

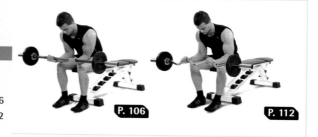

Rowing

Here are the main goals of this circuit:
- Strengthen the biceps and the long head of the triceps so that you can row powerfully for long periods.
- Strengthen the forearm flexors so that you can keep the oars firmly in your grasp.

Repeat at least 2 times per week.

Do this circuit 2 or 3 times in a row taking as little rest time as possible between sets.

- Pull-up   P. 85
  30 to 20 repetitions0
- Triceps–back combo with a high pulley   P. 138
  20 to 15 repetitions
- Reverse curl with a bar   P. 104
  25 to 15 repetitions
- Wrist curl   P. 106
  30 to 20 repetitions

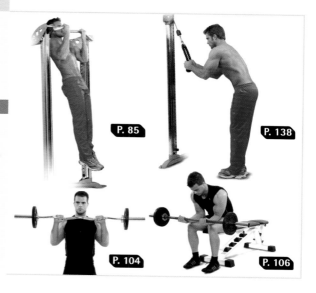

169

Kayaking and Sailing

Here are the main goals of this circuit:
– Strengthen the biceps.
– Strengthen the long head of the triceps.
– Strengthen the gripping strength in your fingers.

Repeat at least once per week.

Do this circuit 2 or 3 times in a row with as little rest time as possible between sets.

- **Pull-up** — P. 85
  20 to 15 repetitions
- **Triceps–back combo with a high pulley** — P. 138
  15 to 8 repetitions
- **Reverse curl with a bar** — P. 104
  20 to 10 repetitions
- **Hanging from a pull-up bar** — P. 141
  30 to 20 repetitions

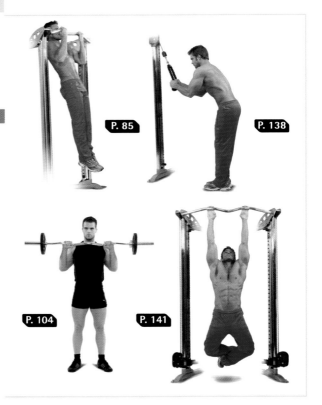

Climbing

Here are the main goals of this circuit:
– Strengthen the biceps.
– Strengthen the entire forearm.
– Strengthen the power in the fingers.

Repeat at least once per week.

Do this circuit 2 or 3 times in a row with as little rest time as possible between sets.

- **Pull-up** — P. 85
  30 to 20 repetitions
- **Reverse curl with a bar** — P. 104
  20 to 10 repetitions
- **Standing wrist curl** — P. 106
  30 to 20 repetitions
- **Hanging from a pull-up bar** — P. 141
  30 to 20 repetitions

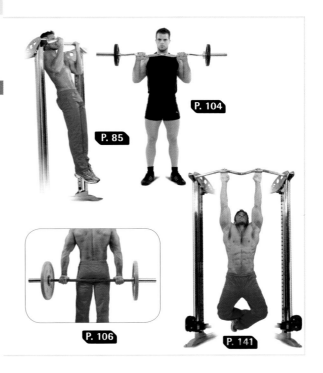

Arm Wrestling

Here are the main goals of this circuit:
- Strengthen the arm flexors.
- Strengthen the entire forearm.
- Strengthen the wrist.

Repeat 2 or 3 times per week.

Between sets, take 1 to 2 minutes to rest.

- Hammer curl   P. 92
  4 or 5 sets of 8 to 6 repetitions
- Reverse curl with a bar   P. 104
  4 or 5 sets of 12 to 10 repetitions
- Pronosupination with a bar   P. 146
  4 or 5 sets of 30 to 20 repetitions
- Standing wrist curl   P. 106
  4 or 5 sets of 15 to 10 repetitions

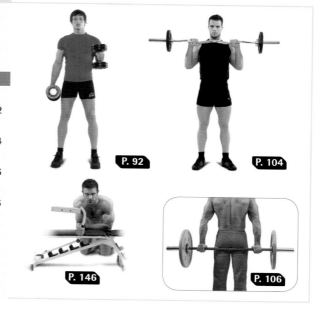

Powerlifting Program for the Bench Press

Here are the main goals of this circuit:
- Increase the power of the triceps.
- Increase the strength of the wrist to guarantee good transmission of arm strength to the bar.

Repeat at least 1 time per week.

Between sets, take 3 to 5 minutes to rest, except for the final superset, which is done with only 30 seconds of rest between sets.

- Narrow-grip bench press with bands   P. 124
  3 or 4 sets of 6 to 3 repetitions
- Partial bench press with bands   P. 124
  3 or 4 sets of 4 to 1 repetitions
- Weighted dip   P. 126
  3 or 4 sets of 6 to 4 repetitions
- Hammer curl   P. 92
  2 or 3 sets of 8 to 6 repetitions

  End the workout with 2 or 3 circuits of 12 to 8 repetitions:
- Wrist curl   P. 106
- Wrist extension   P. 112

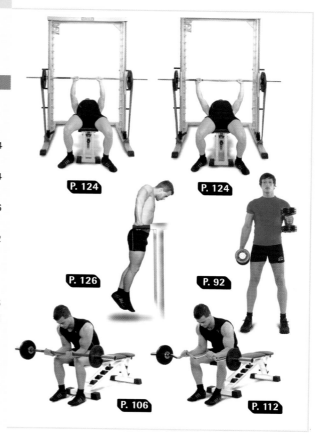

Exercise Index

Library of Congress Cataloging-in-Publication Data

Delavier, Frédéric.
  [Guide de musculation des bras. English]
  Delavier's anatomy for bigger, stronger arms / Frédéric Delavier, Michael Gundill.
      p. cm.
  Includes index.
  ISBN 978-1-4504-4021-9 (soft cover) -- ISBN 1-4504-4021-5 (soft cover)
  1. Arm--Muscles. 2. Muscle strength. 3. Weight training. I. Gundill, Michael. II. Title. III. Title: Anatomy for bigger, stronger arms.
  QM165.D4513 2012
  611'.73--dc23
                         2012013485

ISBN-10: 1-4504-4021-5 (print)
ISBN-13: 978-1-4504-4021-9 (print)

Copyright © 2011 by Éditions Vigot, 23 rue de l'École de Médecine, 75006 Paris, France

This publication is written and published to provide accurate and authoritative information relevant to the subject matter presented. It is published and sold with the understanding that the author and publisher are not engaged in rendering legal, medical, or other professional services by reason of their authorship or publication of this work. If medical or other expert assistance is required, the services of a competent professional person should be sought.

This book is a revised edition of *Guide de Musculation des Bras*, published in 2011 by Éditions Vigot.

Photography: © All rights reserved
Illustrations: © All illustrations by Frédéric Delavier
Main model: David Kimmerle
Modeling and design: Graph'm
Editing: Sophie Lilienfeld

Human Kinetics books are available at special discounts for bulk purchase. Special editions or book excerpts can also be created to specification. For details, contact the Special Sales Manager at Human Kinetics.

Printed in France - L61529   10   9   8   7   6   5   4   3   2   1

Human Kinetics
Website: www.HumanKinetics.com

United States: Human Kinetics
P.O. Box 5076
Champaign, IL 61825-5076
800-747-4457
e-mail: humank@hkusa.com

Canada: Human Kinetics
475 Devonshire Road Unit 100
Windsor, ON N8Y 2L5
800-465-7301 (in Canada only)
e-mail: info@hkcanada.com

Europe: Human Kinetics
107 Bradford Road
Stanningley
Leeds LS28 6AT, United Kingdom
+44 (0) 113 255 5665
e-mail: hk@hkeurope.com

Australia: Human Kinetics
57A Price Avenue
Lower Mitcham, South Australia 5062
08 8372 0999
e-mail: info@hkaustralia.com

New Zealand: Human Kinetics
P.O. Box 80
Torrens Park, South Australia 5062
0800 222 062
e-mail: info@hknewzealand.com

E5806